KIDNEY DISEASE RECIPES FOR NEWLY DIAGNOSED

The Ultimate Complete Guide for Nutritious Renal Diet to be in charge of Kidney disease and be a dialysis free patient

Elizabeth D. Marlow

Copyright© [2024] by [**Elizabeth D. Marlow**]

All rights reserved. No part of this book may be reproduced, distributed, or transmitted in any form or by any means, including photocopying, recording, or other electronic or mechanical methods, without the prior written permission of the publisher, except in the case of brief quotations embodied in critical reviews and certain other noncommercial uses permitted by copyright law.

Table of contents

INTRODUCTION

Why another kidney disease diet or meal planning book?

As you hold this book in your hands or scroll through its pages, you might be wondering, "Why another kidney disease diet or meal planning book?" It's a legitimate question, and one we believe deserves a comprehensive answer. After all, your journey towards managing kidney disease is a profoundly personal and transformative one, and it's crucial to understand the purpose and value of this resource.

The Landscape of Kidney Disease

Kidney disease is a pervasive health concern that affects millions of individuals worldwide. Its impact is not just physical but extends into emotional, social, and lifestyle aspects of a person's life. The journey through kidney disease is marked by uncertainty, medical challenges, dietary restrictions, and profound lifestyle adjustments. It's a path that no one chooses, but many must navigate.

In this landscape, countless resources have been dedicated to helping individuals like you manage their kidney health. Existing books, articles, websites, and medical advice abound. These resources have undoubtedly been invaluable to countless individuals, offering guidance, knowledge, and support.

However, the evolving nature of medicine and nutrition, coupled with the uniqueness of each person's experience, leads us to the conclusion that there is room for another book on this subject – a book designed to address specific aspects and aspirations of those who are newly diagnosed with kidney disease.

The Power of Updated Information

One compelling reason for a new addition to the library of kidney disease resources is the ever-advancing field of medical knowledge. Researchers, doctors, and nutritionists continuously study kidney disease, seeking to uncover more effective treatment approaches, refine dietary recommendations, and improve the quality of life for patients.

This book strives to offer you the most current information available. It serves as a bridge between the latest research findings and your daily life. By staying up-to-date with the most recent developments, we can provide you with the tools to make informed decisions about your health and well-being.

A Personalized Approach to Kidney Health

Kidney disease is a highly individualized condition. No two people will experience it in exactly the same way. Therefore, the "one-size-fits-all" approach may not suffice. This book seeks to offer a personalized perspective on managing kidney disease through diet and lifestyle.

By presenting a diverse range of dietary options, recipes, and strategies, we aim to cater to various tastes, preferences, and cultural backgrounds. We understand that adhering to a renal diet can be challenging, and our goal is to make it as manageable and enjoyable as possible.

Culinary Creativity and Nutritional Balance

A key aspect of living well with kidney disease is embracing culinary creativity while maintaining a delicate nutritional balance. Many individuals mistakenly assume that a renal diet means bland and tasteless meals. This couldn't be further from the truth.

Within the pages of this book, you'll discover a treasure trove of kidney-friendly recipes that tantalize your taste buds while adhering to dietary restrictions. We believe that food should be a source of joy, even when managing a medical condition.

Inspiration and Empowerment

Beyond dietary recommendations, this book aims to inspire and empower you to take control of your kidney health journey. You are not defined by your diagnosis, but rather by your resilience, determination, and ability to adapt and thrive.

Throughout these chapters, you'll find not only practical advice but also stories of individuals who have faced kidney disease with courage and grace. Their experiences will serve as a source of motivation, reminding you that you are not alone on this path.

The Accessibility of Knowledge

Finally, we recognize that different resources resonate with different individuals. This book adds another voice to the chorus of existing materials, providing an alternative perspective that may resonate with you on a personal level. We aim to be a source of support and guidance for those who may not have found the information they seek in other publications.

This book is not merely another entry in the realm of kidney disease literature; it is a reflection of our commitment to your well-being. It is an invitation to embark on a journey toward improved kidney health, a dialysis-free future, and a life filled with vitality and purpose. We hope that within these pages, you will find the

Chapter 1

Understanding Kidney Disease

The kidneys, those unassuming bean-shaped organs nestled within our abdominal cavities, perform an extraordinary and often underappreciated role in maintaining our overall health. These two small powerhouses filter waste products and excess fluids from the bloodstream, regulate blood pressure, balance electrolytes, and produce essential hormones. Yet, when kidney function becomes compromised, it can lead to a complex and potentially life-altering condition known as kidney disease.

What is Kidney Disease?

Kidney disease, medically known as renal disease or nephropathy, is a complex and potentially debilitating condition characterized by the gradual or sudden deterioration of kidney function. The kidneys are paired, bean-shaped organs located in the abdominal cavity, and they perform vital roles in maintaining the body's internal equilibrium.

These remarkable organs are responsible for filtering waste products and excess fluids from the bloodstream, a process that helps regulate electrolytes, fluid volume, and blood pressure. The kidneys also produce essential hormones, such as erythropoietin, which stimulates the production of red blood cells, and renin, which plays a crucial role in blood pressure regulation.

Kidney disease can manifest in various forms, and its severity can range from mild to severe. Common causes of kidney disease include diabetes, high blood pressure, certain medications, infections, genetic factors, and autoimmune conditions. It is a pervasive health issue, affecting millions of individuals globally, and its prevalence continues to rise.

One of the defining features of kidney disease is its ability to progress silently, often with few noticeable symptoms, especially in its early stages. This silent progression is why it is often referred to as a "silent killer." Without regular medical check-ups and screening, individuals may remain unaware of their kidney condition until significant damage has occurred.

Early detection and comprehensive understanding of kidney disease are essential for effective management and intervention. In subsequent chapters, we will explore the various types of kidney disease, the risk factors associated with its development, and practical steps individuals can take to maintain and enhance their kidney health.

Types of Kidney Disease

Kidney disease encompasses a range of disorders that affect the kidneys' structure and function. These disorders can be broadly categorised into several types, each with its unique causes, characteristics, and implications. Here are some of the most common types of kidney disease:

Chronic Kidney Disease (CKD): This is a progressive condition where kidney function gradually deteriorates over an extended period. It often develops slowly and may go unnoticed in its early stages. CKD is typically classified into five stages, with stage 1 being the mildest and stage 5 indicating end-stage renal disease (ESRD), where kidney function is severely impaired.

Acute Kidney Injury (AKI): Acute Kidney Injury is a sudden and often reversible decline in kidney function. It typically occurs over a short period and is often caused by factors like infections, medications, severe dehydration, or trauma. Timely medical intervention can lead to a full recovery in cases of AKI.

Polycystic Kidney Disease (PKD): PKD is a genetic disorder characterized by the growth of numerous fluid-filled cysts within the kidneys. Over time, these cysts can enlarge, leading to kidney enlargement and a decline in function. PKD can cause both acute and chronic kidney issues.

Glomerulonephritis: This term refers to inflammation of the glomeruli, which are tiny blood vessels within the kidneys responsible for filtering the blood. Glomerulonephritis can be acute or chronic and is often caused by immune system disorders, infections, or other underlying health conditions.

Diabetic Nephropathy: Diabetic nephropathy is a specific type of kidney disease that arises as a complication of uncontrolled diabetes. High blood sugar levels can damage the small blood vessels in the kidneys, leading to impaired kidney function over time.

Hypertensive Nephropathy: Hypertensive nephropathy results from long-term, uncontrolled high blood pressure. The persistent strain on the kidneys' blood vessels can lead to kidney damage and reduced function.

Nephrotic Syndrome: Nephrotic syndrome is characterized by the leakage of large amounts of protein into the urine, leading to swelling, high cholesterol levels, and increased susceptibility to infections. It can result from various underlying kidney conditions.

Kidney Stones: While not a type of kidney disease per se, kidney stones are common and can cause severe pain and potential kidney damage if left untreated. They are crystalline structures that form in the urinary tract and can obstruct the flow of urine.

These are just a few examples of the various types of kidney disease. Each type may require different approaches to management and treatment, making it crucial for individuals to receive an accurate diagnosis and personalized care based on their specific condition. Early detection and understanding of the underlying causes are essential for effectively managing kidney disease and preserving kidney function.

Reason for kidney disease

Kidney disease can result from a variety of causes and risk factors. Understanding these reasons is crucial for both prevention and early detection. Here are some of the primary reasons for kidney disease:

1. Diabetes: Diabetes is one of the leading causes of kidney disease. High blood sugar levels over an extended period can damage the small blood vessels in the kidneys, leading to

kidney damage and impaired function. This condition is known as diabetic nephropathy.

2. Hypertension (High Blood Pressure): Uncontrolled high blood pressure can put excessive strain on the blood vessels in the kidneys. Over time, this can lead to kidney damage and reduced function, a condition known as hypertensive nephropathy.

3. Glomerulonephritis: Glomerulonephritis is characterized by inflammation of the glomeruli, which are the tiny filtering units within the kidneys. It can be caused by immune system disorders, infections, or other underlying health conditions.

4. Polycystic Kidney Disease (PKD): PKD is a genetic disorder characterized by the growth of numerous fluid-filled cysts within the kidneys. These cysts can enlarge over time, leading to kidney enlargement and a decline in function.

5. Infections: Certain infections, such as urinary tract infections (UTIs) and kidney infections, can directly affect kidney function if left untreated or if they become chronic.

6. Autoimmune Diseases: Conditions like lupus, rheumatoid arthritis, and other autoimmune disorders can cause inflammation in various parts of the body, including the kidneys. This chronic inflammation can lead to kidney damage.

7. Medications: Some medications, when used long-term and in high doses, can harm the kidneys. Nonsteroidal anti-inflammatory drugs (NSAIDs), certain antibiotics, and certain blood pressure medications are examples of drugs that can affect kidney function.

8. Kidney Stones: The formation of kidney stones, crystalline structures that develop in the urinary tract, can lead to kidney damage if the stones obstruct the flow of urine or cause repeated infections.

9. Heredity: Family history can play a role in kidney disease risk. Some kidney conditions, like PKD, are hereditary, meaning they can be passed down through generations.

10. Obesity: Excess body weight, particularly obesity, is associated with an increased risk of developing kidney disease. Obesity can contribute to conditions like diabetes and hypertension, both of which are risk factors for kidney disease.

11. Smoking: Smoking can damage blood vessels, including those in the kidneys, potentially leading to reduced kidney function over time.

12. Age: The risk of kidney disease tends to increase with age, as kidney function naturally declines as part of the aging process.

Understanding these reasons for kidney disease is essential for preventive measures and early detection. Regular medical check-ups, monitoring of blood pressure and blood sugar levels, and lifestyle modifications can help reduce the risk and manage kidney disease effectively.

Chapter 2

Kidney-Friendly Nutrition Basics

Proper nutrition is the cornerstone of managing kidney disease effectively. A kidney-friendly diet can help alleviate symptoms, slow disease progression, and improve overall well-being. In this chapter, we will explore the fundamentals of kidney-friendly nutrition to empower you with the knowledge needed to make informed dietary choices.

Understanding Dietary Restrictions

A renal diet is designed to minimize the strain on your kidneys by controlling the intake of certain nutrients. Key components to monitor include:

1. **Protein**:
Why It Matters: Protein metabolism produces waste products that the kidneys must filter.

Reducing protein intake can lessen the burden on these vital organs.

What to Do: Your healthcare provider will recommend an appropriate daily protein limit. High-quality protein sources like lean meats, poultry, fish, and eggs are preferred. Plant-based proteins like tofu and legumes are also good options.

2. **Sodium** (Salt):

Why It Matters: Excess sodium can lead to fluid retention and elevated blood pressure, both of which can strain the kidneys.

What to Do: Limit salt intake by avoiding processed foods, canned soups, and restaurant meals. Opt for fresh, unprocessed foods and use herbs and spices for flavor.

3. **Potassium**:

Why It Matters: High potassium levels can disrupt heart rhythms and pose risks to kidney function.

What to Do: Limit potassium-rich foods like bananas, oranges, potatoes, and tomatoes.

Cooking techniques such as boiling or leaching can reduce potassium content in certain foods.

4. Phosphorus:

Why It Matters: Elevated phosphorus levels can weaken bones and contribute to cardiovascular issues in kidney disease.

What to Do: Limit phosphorus-rich foods like dairy products, nuts, and processed foods. Phosphorus binders may be prescribed to control phosphorus absorption.

5. Fluids:

Why It Matters: Kidneys may lose their ability to regulate fluid balance as kidney disease progresses. Excessive fluid intake can lead to fluid retention and swelling.

What to Do: Monitor daily fluid intake according to your healthcare provider's recommendations. Be mindful of foods with high water content, like fruits and vegetables.

Creating a Kidney-Friendly Meal Plan

A well-balanced meal plan is essential for managing kidney disease effectively. Here are some key considerations:

1. **Portion Control**:
Why It Matters: Managing portion sizes can help control nutrient intake and prevent overloading your kidneys.

What to Do: Use measuring cups and scales to monitor portion sizes. Aim for balanced meals that include appropriate portions of protein, carbohydrates, and healthy fats.

2. **Nutrient Balance**:
Why It Matters: Balancing nutrients is crucial for overall health and energy levels.

What to Do: Incorporate a variety of foods to ensure a diverse nutrient intake. Consult with a registered dietitian to create a personalized meal plan that suits your specific dietary needs.

3. **Cooking Methods**:

Why It Matters: Cooking methods can affect the nutritional content of foods.

What to Do: Choose cooking methods like baking, grilling, steaming, and boiling to preserve nutrients and limit added fats and salt.

4. **Food Labels**:

Why It Matters: Reading food labels helps identify hidden sodium and phosphorus in packaged foods.

What to Do: Pay close attention to nutrition labels and look for low-sodium and low-phosphorus options. Choose products with less than 20% of the daily value for sodium per serving.

Importance of Nutrient Balance

Nutrient balance is of paramount importance for overall health and well-being. Achieving a proper balance of essential nutrients in your diet ensures that your body functions optimally and can have a significant impact on various aspects of your health. Here's why nutrient balance is crucial:

1. Optimal Health: Nutrient balance ensures that your body receives all the essential vitamins, minerals, proteins, carbohydrates, and fats it needs to function correctly. Each nutrient plays a unique role in supporting bodily functions, from energy production to immune system health.

2. Energy Production: Carbohydrates, fats, and proteins are macronutrients that provide energy for daily activities. Maintaining a balance of these nutrients ensures you have the necessary energy to perform tasks, exercise, and stay active.

3. Metabolism Regulation: Nutrients like vitamins and minerals are crucial for regulating metabolic processes. They act as coenzymes or cofactors in various enzymatic reactions that control energy metabolism, hormone production, and the breakdown of nutrients for energy.

4. Tissue Repair and Growth: Adequate protein intake is essential for tissue repair and growth, whether you're recovering from an injury, building muscle, or supporting the body's natural repair processes.

5. Immune System Function: Vitamins and minerals, such as vitamin C, vitamin D, and zinc, play vital roles in supporting immune system function. A well-balanced diet ensures your immune system has the nutrients it needs to protect you from illnesses and infections.

6. Heart Health: Maintaining a balanced intake of healthy fats, such as monounsaturated and polyunsaturated fats, can help lower the risk of heart disease by improving cholesterol levels and reducing inflammation.

7. Blood Sugar Control: Proper nutrient balance, especially in carbohydrates, helps regulate blood sugar levels. This is particularly important for individuals with conditions like diabetes.

8. Bone Health: Adequate intake of calcium and vitamin D is crucial for maintaining strong and

healthy bones. Nutrient balance supports bone density and can reduce the risk of conditions like osteoporosis.

9. Weight Management: Achieving a balance between calorie intake and energy expenditure is key to weight management. Nutrient-dense foods that provide essential nutrients while keeping calorie intake in check can help maintain a healthy weight.

10. Digestive Health: Fiber, a type of carbohydrate found in plant-based foods, promotes digestive health by preventing constipation, improving gut bacteria balance, and supporting overall gut health.

11. Mental Well-being: Nutrient balance can also have an impact on mental health. Certain nutrients, such as omega-3 fatty acids and B vitamins, are associated with improved mood and cognitive function.

12. Disease Prevention: A balanced diet rich in essential nutrients can help reduce the risk of chronic diseases like diabetes, cardiovascular disease, and certain types of cancer.

Achieving nutrient balance in your diet involves consuming a variety of foods from different food groups to ensure you receive a wide range of nutrients. Consulting with a registered dietitian can provide personalized guidance on how to achieve and maintain nutrient balance while considering individual dietary needs and health goals.

Monitoring Fluid Intake

Monitoring fluid intake is crucial for individuals with kidney disease, as the kidneys may lose their ability to regulate fluid balance as the condition progresses. Proper fluid management helps prevent complications like fluid retention and electrolyte imbalances. Here are some essential tips for monitoring and managing fluid intake:

1. Know Your Recommended Fluid Limit: Work with your healthcare provider or registered dietitian to determine your daily fluid intake limit. This limit is based on factors such as the stage of kidney disease, age, body size, and individual health needs.

2. Track Fluid Intake: Keep a daily record of your fluid intake, including water, beverages, and even moisture-rich foods like soups, fruits, and vegetables. Using a journal or smartphone app can help you track your intake accurately.

3. Measure Fluids: Use standard measuring cups or a kitchen scale to measure your beverages and fluids. This ensures you have an accurate record of how much you're consuming.

4. Set a Fluid Schedule: Establish a structured schedule for fluid consumption throughout the day. This can help you distribute your intake evenly and avoid excessive thirst.

5. Be Mindful of High-Water Foods: Some foods, like watermelon, cucumbers, and oranges, have a high water content. Be aware of these foods and factor their water content into your daily limit.

6. Limit High-Sodium Foods: High-sodium foods can increase thirst and make it more challenging to adhere to your fluid limit. Avoid

or minimize processed foods, canned soups, and salty snacks.

7. Use Smaller Glasses or Cups: Serving fluids in smaller glasses or cups can help you manage portion sizes and avoid excessive intake.

8. Practice Thirst Management: Instead of drinking fluids as soon as you feel thirsty, try to manage your thirst. Swishing and spitting out water, chewing gum, or sucking on ice chips can help alleviate thirst without increasing fluid intake.

9. Monitor Urine Output: Pay attention to your urine output and color. Dark or concentrated urine may indicate dehydration, while frequent, pale urine may suggest you are well-hydrated.

10. Engage Your Healthcare Team: Regularly communicate with your healthcare provider and registered dietitian about your fluid management efforts. They can help you make adjustments to your fluid intake based on your specific health status.

11. Stay Informed: Continuously educate yourself about the fluids in different foods and beverages. This knowledge can help you make informed choices and avoid hidden sources of excessive fluid intake.

12. Consider Individual Needs: Recognize that fluid needs can vary from person to person. Factors like climate, physical activity level, and medications may influence your specific fluid requirements.

Managing fluid intake can be challenging, but it is a crucial aspect of kidney disease management. By diligently monitoring your fluid intake, adhering to your prescribed limits, and working closely with your healthcare team, you can maintain proper fluid balance, reduce the risk of complications, and support your overall kidney health.

Essential Nutrients for Kidney Health

Maintaining kidney health relies on consuming essential nutrients that support kidney function and overall well-being. Here are key nutrients that play a crucial role in kidney health:

1. Protein: Adequate protein intake is important for tissue repair and overall health. However, for individuals with kidney disease, protein intake may need to be controlled and tailored to their specific needs. It's essential to work with a healthcare provider or dietitian to determine the appropriate protein level for your condition.

2. Fluids: Monitoring fluid intake is vital for kidney health, especially in cases of kidney disease. Restricting fluid intake as recommended by your healthcare provider helps manage fluid balance and prevent complications like fluid retention and high blood pressure.

3. Sodium (Salt): Limiting sodium intake is crucial for controlling blood pressure and reducing the risk of fluid retention. Avoiding

processed foods, canned soups, and high-sodium condiments can help lower sodium intake.

4. Potassium: Managing potassium intake is essential, as high potassium levels can disrupt heart rhythms and pose risks to kidney function. Limiting potassium-rich foods like bananas, oranges, potatoes, and tomatoes is often necessary.

5. Phosphorus: Keeping phosphorus levels in check is essential to support kidney health. High phosphorus levels can weaken bones and contribute to cardiovascular issues. Restricting phosphorus-rich foods like dairy products and processed foods is typically recommended.

6. Calcium: Adequate calcium intake is necessary for strong bones. However, individuals with kidney disease may need to monitor calcium intake, especially if they are prescribed phosphorus binders, which can affect calcium absorption.

7. Vitamin D: Vitamin D is essential for calcium absorption and bone health. Many people with

kidney disease have lower levels of active vitamin D, so supplements may be necessary under medical supervision.

8. Vitamin B Complex: B vitamins, including B6, B9 (folate), and B12, are important for various bodily functions, including red blood cell production and nerve health. Kidney disease can affect vitamin B metabolism, so monitoring levels and supplementation may be required.

9. Iron: Adequate iron intake is crucial for preventing anemia. However, individuals with kidney disease may require special consideration regarding iron supplements, as kidney function affects iron utilization.

10. Omega-3 Fatty Acids: Omega-3 fatty acids found in fatty fish, flaxseeds, and walnuts have anti-inflammatory properties and can support cardiovascular health, which is important for individuals with kidney disease.

11. Antioxidants: Antioxidants, such as vitamins C and E, can help protect cells from damage and support overall health. Including

antioxidant-rich foods in your diet can be beneficial.

12. Fiber: Fiber from fruits, vegetables, and whole grains helps maintain digestive health and may assist in managing blood sugar levels, which is important for individuals with kidney disease, especially those with diabetes.

Balancing these essential nutrients in your diet is crucial for maintaining kidney health. However, it's important to note that the specific dietary recommendations can vary depending on the stage of kidney disease, individual needs, and underlying conditions. Always consult with your healthcare provider or a registered dietitian who specializes in renal nutrition to create a personalized dietary plan tailored to your unique circumstances.

Healthy Fats

Healthy fats are a crucial component of a balanced diet and play a vital role in supporting overall health. These fats provide essential fatty acids, aid in nutrient absorption, and offer a source of long-lasting energy. Incorporating healthy fats into your diet can have a positive impact on your well-being. Here are some examples of healthy fats and their benefits:

1. Monounsaturated Fats:
Sources: Olive oil, avocados, nuts (e.g., almonds, peanuts, cashews), seeds (e.g., sunflower seeds), and certain fruits (e.g., olives).

Benefits: Monounsaturated fats are heart-healthy and can help reduce LDL (low-density lipoprotein) cholesterol levels, which is known as "bad" cholesterol. They also provide a source of vitamin E, an antioxidant.

2. Polyunsaturated Fats:
Sources: Fatty fish (e.g., salmon, mackerel, trout), flaxseeds, chia seeds, walnuts, soybean oil, and corn oil.

Benefits: Polyunsaturated fats are rich in essential omega-3 and omega-6 fatty acids. Omega-3 fatty acids, in particular, support heart health, reduce inflammation, and may improve cognitive function.

3. Omega-3 Fatty Acids:
Sources: Fatty fish (e.g., salmon, mackerel, sardines), flaxseeds, chia seeds, walnuts, hemp seeds, and algae-based supplements.

Benefits: Omega-3 fatty acids are associated with a lower risk of heart disease, improved brain health, and reduced inflammation. They are essential for maintaining healthy cell membranes and brain function.

4. Avocado: Avocado is a unique fruit that is rich in healthy monounsaturated fats. It also provides fiber, vitamins (such as folate and vitamin K), and minerals.

5. Nuts and Seeds: Nuts and seeds are nutrient-dense sources of healthy fats, protein, fiber, vitamins, and minerals. They make for satisfying and nutritious snacks.

6. Olive Oil: Extra virgin olive oil is a staple of the Mediterranean diet and is renowned for its heart-healthy monounsaturated fats and antioxidants.

7. Fatty Fish: Fatty fish like salmon, mackerel, and trout are excellent sources of omega-3 fatty acids, which support cardiovascular health and brain function.

8. Coconut: Coconut products, including coconut oil and coconut milk, contain medium-chain triglycerides (MCTs), which can provide a quick source of energy and may have potential health benefits.

9. Dark Chocolate: High-quality dark chocolate with a high cocoa content (70% or more) contains healthy fats, antioxidants, and may have heart-protective effects when consumed in moderation.

It's important to remember that while healthy fats offer numerous benefits, they are calorie-dense, so portion control is key, especially if you're looking to manage your weight. Replacing saturated and trans fats with healthy fats can contribute to better overall health. Aim to include a variety of these healthy fat sources in your diet to enjoy their nutritional advantages while supporting your well-being.

How Much is Too Much Protein

Consuming too much protein can have both short-term and long-term health implications. The optimal daily protein intake varies depending on factors like age, sex, activity level, and overall health. However, it's important to understand when protein intake becomes excessive and the potential risks associated with overconsumption.

Here are some considerations regarding how much protein is "too much":

1. Exceeding Daily Needs: In general, a balanced diet typically includes protein intake that ranges from 10% to 35% of total daily calories. Consuming protein within this range is considered appropriate for most individuals.

2. Kidney Strain: Excessive protein intake can strain the kidneys, particularly in individuals with preexisting kidney conditions. The kidneys are responsible for filtering waste products generated during protein metabolism, and over time, high protein intake can increase the workload on these organs.

3. Dehydration: A diet high in protein may lead to increased water loss through urine. This can potentially contribute to dehydration, especially if an individual doesn't increase their fluid intake to compensate.

4. Calcium Loss: High-protein diets may result in increased calcium excretion in the urine, potentially leading to negative impacts on bone health over time. Adequate calcium intake is crucial for maintaining strong bones.

5. Digestive Issues: Some people may experience digestive discomfort, such as bloating or constipation, when consuming excessive protein. This can be due to insufficient fiber intake or an imbalance in nutrient ratios.

6. Potential for Weight Gain: While protein is essential for various bodily functions, excessive protein intake alone does not necessarily promote weight loss. Consuming more calories, regardless of their source, can lead to weight gain if they exceed your daily energy needs.

7. Potential for Nutrient Imbalances: Focusing solely on high-protein foods may lead to nutrient imbalances, as other essential nutrients from fruits, vegetables, and grains may be lacking in the diet.

8. Long-Term Health Implications: Some studies suggest that chronic high-protein intake, particularly from animal sources, may be associated with an increased risk of certain health conditions, such as heart disease and certain types of cancer.

It's essential to strike a balance in your protein intake that aligns with your individual health goals and dietary needs. Consulting with a registered dietitian or healthcare provider can help you determine the appropriate protein intake for your specific circumstances. Factors such as age, activity level, muscle mass, and underlying health conditions should be considered when determining your protein needs to ensure you are not consuming too much protein on a regular basis.

Chapter 3

Meal Planning for Kidney Health

Meal planning for kidney health is essential to ensure that you meet your nutritional needs while managing the dietary restrictions associated with kidney disease. Here are some guidelines for creating a kidney-friendly meal plan:

1. Consult with a Dietitian: Start by consulting with a registered dietitian who specializes in renal nutrition. They can provide personalized guidance based on your specific kidney disease stage, dietary preferences, and health goals.

2. Determine Your Nutritional Needs: Work with your dietitian to determine your daily requirements for calories, protein, sodium, potassium, phosphorus, and fluids. These values will serve as the foundation for your meal plan.

3. Balance Protein Intake: Protein is essential for health, but in kidney disease, excessive protein intake can be harmful. Follow your

prescribed daily protein limit while ensuring you get enough high-quality protein from sources like lean meats, poultry, fish, and plant-based options like tofu and legumes.

4. Control Sodium Intake: Limit sodium (salt) by avoiding processed foods, canned soups, and restaurant meals. Use herbs, spices, lemon juice, and vinegar for flavor instead of salt.

5. Manage Potassium: Monitor potassium intake by limiting high-potassium foods like bananas, oranges, tomatoes, and potatoes. Cooking techniques like boiling or leaching can help reduce potassium content in certain foods.

6. Limit Phosphorus: Restrict phosphorus-rich foods like dairy products, nuts, seeds, and processed foods. Take phosphorus binders as prescribed to control phosphorus absorption.

7. Watch Fluid Intake: Monitor and restrict fluid intake as recommended by your healthcare provider to manage fluid balance and prevent complications like fluid retention and high blood pressure.

8. Plan Balanced Meals: Create well-balanced meals that include appropriate portions of protein, carbohydrates, and healthy fats. Include a variety of fruits and vegetables, emphasizing those lower in potassium.

9. Choose Kidney-Friendly Snacks: Opt for kidney-friendly snacks like apple slices, cucumber slices, or small servings of low-potassium fruits. Avoid high-sodium or high-phosphorus snacks.

10. Cooking Methods: Use cooking methods like baking, grilling, steaming, and boiling to preserve nutrients and limit added fats and salt.

11. Monitor Food Labels: Read food labels carefully to identify hidden sodium and phosphorus in packaged foods. Look for products labeled as "low sodium" or "phosphorus-free" when applicable.

12. Portion Control: Measure and control portion sizes to manage nutrient intake effectively and avoid overconsumption.

13. Limit High-Potassium Condiments: Be cautious with high-potassium condiments like soy sauce and ketchup. Opt for alternatives with lower potassium content.

14. Stay Hydrated: Follow your prescribed fluid intake while accounting for the fluids in foods like soups, fruits, and vegetables.

15. Track Progress: Maintain a food diary to track your meals, fluid intake, and symptoms. Share this information with your healthcare team to make necessary adjustments to your meal plan.

16. Individualize Your Plan: Remember that dietary needs vary from person to person, so your meal plan should be tailored to your specific circumstances and preferences.

Consistent adherence to a kidney-friendly meal plan, along with regular communication with your healthcare team, can help manage kidney disease effectively, slow its progression, and support your overall well-being.

Creating a Kidney-Friendly Meal Plan

Daily Meal Planning

Daily meal planning for kidney health involves careful consideration of your dietary restrictions and nutritional requirements. Here's a sample daily meal plan to help you get started:

Breakfast:
- Scrambled eggs with spinach (low in potassium) and a sprinkle of low-phosphorus cheese.
- Whole-grain toast (choose a lower-sodium variety).
- Sliced strawberries (a low-potassium fruit).
- A small glass of apple juice (limit portion size to manage fluid intake).

Mid-Morning Snack:
- A handful of unsalted almonds or walnuts.
- A serving of crisp, low-potassium veggies like cucumber or bell peppers.

Lunch:

- Grilled chicken breast or tofu (for protein) with a light seasoning of herbs and lemon.
- A side of steamed asparagus (a low-potassium vegetable).
- Quinoa or brown rice (a whole grain).
- A mixed green salad with a vinaigrette dressing (homemade to control sodium).

Afternoon Snack:

- Greek yogurt or a dairy-free alternative (look for lower-phosphorus options).
- Sliced peaches (canned peaches in juice, drained, can be a low-potassium choice).

Dinner:

- Baked salmon (rich in omega-3 fatty acids) with a squeeze of lemon.
- Mashed cauliflower (a lower-potassium alternative to potatoes).
- Steamed green beans or broccoli (low-potassium vegetables).
- A small roll or breadstick (choose one lower in sodium).

Evening Snack (if needed):

- A small serving of a low-potassium fruit like apple slices or blueberries.
- A cup of herbal tea (caffeine-free) or plain water.

Notes:

-Be mindful of portion sizes and ensure they align with your prescribed dietary restrictions.

- Limit salt and use herbs, spices, and lemon juice to add flavor to your meals.

- Drink fluids according to your recommended daily limit, including any fluids from foods.

- Adjust the meal plan based on your specific nutritional needs and any guidance from your dietitian or healthcare provider.

Remember that this is just a sample meal plan, and individualized recommendations will vary based on your unique circumstances, including your stage of kidney disease and any comorbidities. Consult with a registered dietitian who specializes in renal nutrition to create a personalized meal plan that suits your specific needs and preferences. Regular communication with your healthcare team is essential for managing kidney disease effectively through dietary choices.

Weekly Meal Prep Tips

Weekly meal prep can be a time-saving and convenient way to ensure you have kidney-friendly meals readily available throughout the week. Here are some tips to help you get started with weekly meal prep for kidney health:

1. Consult with a Dietitian: Before you begin meal prepping, consult with a registered dietitian who specializes in renal nutrition. They can provide personalized guidance based on your dietary restrictions and nutritional needs.

2. Plan Your Meals: Start by creating a weekly meal plan that includes breakfast, lunch, dinner, and snacks. Ensure that each meal aligns with your dietary restrictions for protein, sodium, potassium, phosphorus, and fluid intake.

Consider recipes that are kidney-friendly, and make a list of ingredients you'll need.

3. Choose Kidney-Friendly Recipes:
   Look for kidney-friendly recipes online or in renal diet cookbooks. Focus on recipes that use fresh, whole ingredients and limit processed or high-sodium foods.

4. Shop Smart: Use your meal plan to create a shopping list. Stick to the list to avoid buying unnecessary items. Choose fresh fruits and vegetables that are in season and fit your dietary restrictions.

5. Prep Ingredients: Wash, chop, and portion vegetables, fruits, and other ingredients for the week. This makes it easier to assemble meals quickly. Pre-cook grains like brown rice or quinoa and store them in portioned containers.

6. Cook in Batches: Prepare larger batches of kidney-friendly proteins like grilled chicken or tofu and store them in separate containers.
Cook a big pot of kidney-friendly soup or stew that can be portioned out for multiple meals.

7. Use Storage Containers: Invest in a variety of reusable, airtight containers in different sizes to store your prepped ingredients and meals. Label containers with the date of preparation to keep track of freshness.

8. Portion Control: When assembling your meals, use a kitchen scale or measuring cups to ensure proper portion sizes according to your dietary restrictions.

9. Freeze Extra Portions: If you've prepared more than you can consume in a week, freeze the extra portions in individual containers. This extends the shelf life of your meals.

10. Plan for Breakfast and Snacks: Don't forget to prepare kidney-friendly breakfast options and snacks, such as boiled eggs, pre-portioned Greek yogurt, or chopped veggies with hummus.

11. Set a Schedule: Designate a specific day and time each week for your meal prep routine. Consistency can make the process more manageable.

Weekly meal prep can simplify your daily routine and help you adhere to your kidney-friendly diet. Regularly review your meal plan and adjust it as needed based on your health and dietary requirements. Meal prep can contribute to better kidney health and overall well-being.

Grocery Shopping for Renal Diet

Smart Food Choices

Making smart food choices is crucial for overall health, especially if you have specific dietary restrictions or health conditions like kidney disease. Here are some tips to help you make wise food choices:

1. Consult a Dietitian: Start by consulting with a registered dietitian who specializes in your specific dietary needs, whether related to kidney health, diabetes, heart health, or any other condition. They can provide personalized guidance.

2. Focus on Whole Foods: Choose whole, minimally processed foods whenever possible. These include fruits, vegetables, whole grains, lean proteins, and healthy fats. Whole foods are often lower in sodium, additives, and preservatives.

3. Read Labels: When buying packaged foods, read nutrition labels carefully. Pay attention to serving sizes, calories, sodium, and other nutrients relevant to your dietary restrictions.

4. Limit Sodium (Salt): Reduce your sodium intake by avoiding highly processed foods, canned soups, and fast food. Opt for low-sodium or no-salt-added versions of products.

5. Choose Lean Proteins: Opt for lean sources of protein, such as skinless poultry, fish, tofu, legumes, and lean cuts of beef or pork. Remove visible fats from meats.

6. Monitor Phosphorus and Potassium: If you have kidney disease, be mindful of foods high in phosphorus and potassium. Your dietitian can provide a list of foods to limit or avoid.

7. Balance Macronutrients: Aim for a balanced diet that includes carbohydrates, protein, and healthy fats. Avoid extreme diets that eliminate entire food groups.

8. Increase Fiber Intake: Include plenty of fiber-rich foods like whole grains, legumes, fruits, and vegetables in your diet. Fiber supports digestive health and helps manage blood sugar levels.

9. Choose Healthy Fats: Opt for sources of healthy fats like olive oil, avocados, nuts, and fatty fish (rich in omega-3 fatty acids). Limit saturated and trans fats found in fried foods and processed snacks.

10. Hydrate Wisely: Stay hydrated, but monitor your fluid intake if you have kidney disease. Sip water throughout the day and consider herbal teas or ice chips as alternatives to quench your thirst.

11. Mindful Eating: Practice mindful eating by savoring each bite, chewing slowly, and paying

attention to hunger and fullness cues. Avoid eating while distracted.

12. Limit Added Sugars: Reduce your intake of foods and beverages high in added sugars, such as sugary drinks, candy, and desserts. Choose naturally sweet options like fruits when you have a sweet craving.

13. Cook at Home: Preparing meals at home allows you to have more control over ingredients and portion sizes. Experiment with kidney-friendly recipes.

14. Plan Ahead: Plan your meals and snacks in advance to ensure that you have kidney-friendly options readily available, especially if you have a busy schedule.

Making smart food choices is an essential part of a healthy lifestyle. It can help you manage your health condition, prevent chronic diseases, and enhance your overall well-being.

Chapter 4

Breakfast Recipes

Here are two kidney-friendly breakfast recipes that are both delicious and suitable for a renal diet:

Oatmeal with Berries and Almonds:

Ingredients:
- 1/2 cup rolled oats (choose low-sodium oats if available)
- 1 cup water or low-potassium milk substitute (such as rice or almond milk)
- 1/4 cup fresh or frozen mixed berries (blueberries, strawberries, raspberries)
- 1 tablespoon chopped almonds (unsalted)
- 1 teaspoon honey or a sugar substitute (if needed)

Instructions:
1. In a saucepan, bring the water or milk to a boil.
2. Stir in the rolled oats and reduce the heat to low. Simmer for about 5 minutes,

stirring occasionally, until the oats are cooked and the mixture thickens.

3. Remove from heat and transfer the oatmeal to a serving bowl.
4. Top with mixed berries and chopped almonds.
5. Drizzle with honey or a sugar substitute for added sweetness if desired.
6. Serve hot and enjoy your kidney-friendly oatmeal breakfast!

Veggie and Cheese Omelette:

Ingredients:
- 2 large eggs (or egg substitute)
- 1/4 cup low-phosphorus cheese (such as mozzarella or Swiss), grated
- 1/4 cup finely chopped bell peppers (choose low-potassium colors like green or yellow)
- 1/4 cup finely chopped spinach (or other low-potassium greens)
- 1/4 cup diced tomatoes (if your dietary restrictions allow)
- Salt and pepper to taste

- Cooking spray or a small amount of olive oil for the pan

Instructions:

1. In a bowl, whisk the eggs until well beaten. Season with a pinch of salt and pepper.
2. Heat a non-stick skillet over medium heat and lightly grease it with cooking spray or a small amount of olive oil.
3. Add the chopped bell peppers and spinach to the skillet and sauté for 2-3 minutes until they begin to soften.
4. Pour the beaten eggs over the sautéed vegetables and allow them to cook without stirring until the edges set.
5. Sprinkle the grated cheese evenly over one half of the omelette.
6. Carefully fold the other half of the omelette over the cheese side.
7. Continue cooking for another 1-2 minutes until the cheese melts, and the omelette is cooked through.
8. Slide the omelette onto a plate, garnish with diced tomatoes (if allowed), and season to taste.

9. Serve hot with a side of kidney-friendly toast or whole-grain bread, if desired.

Apple & Oat Porridge

Ingredients:

- 1/2 cup rolled oats (choose low-sodium oats if available
- 1 cup water or low-potassium milk substitute (such as rice or almond milk)
- 1 small apple, peeled, cored, and chopped into small pieces
- 1/4 teaspoon ground cinnamon
- 1 tablespoon chopped almonds (unsalted, for garnish)
- 1 teaspoon honey or a sugar substitute (if needed)

Instructions:

1. In a saucepan, combine the water or milk substitute, rolled oats, and chopped apple pieces.
2. Sprinkle ground cinnamon over the mixture and stir well.
3. Place the saucepan over medium heat and bring the mixture to a boil.

4. Reduce the heat to low and simmer for about 5-7 minutes, stirring occasionally, until the oats are cooked, and the porridge thickens. If it becomes too thick, you can add a little more liquid to achieve your desired consistency.
5. Remove from heat and transfer the apple and oat porridge to a serving bowl.
6. Drizzle with honey or a sugar substitute for added sweetness if desired.
7. Sprinkle chopped almonds over the top for a crunchy texture and extra flavor.
8. Serve hot and enjoy your kidney-friendly Apple & Oat Porridge!

This wholesome and comforting porridge is a nutritious choice for a kidney-friendly breakfast. It's rich in fiber, vitamins, and minerals, and the addition of apples and cinnamon provides a delightful flavor. Adjust ingredients and portion sizes based on your specific dietary restrictions and recommendations from your healthcare provider or dietitian.

Baked Oatmeal with Berries

Ingredients:

- 1 cup rolled oats (choose low-sodium oats if available)
- 1/4 cup chopped almonds (unsalted)
- 1/4 cup dried cranberries (unsweetened)
- 1/4 cup fresh or frozen mixed berries (blueberries, strawberries, raspberries)
- 1/2 teaspoon ground cinnamon
- 1 1/2 cups low-potassium milk substitute (such as rice or almond milk)
- 2 tablespoons honey or a sugar substitute (if needed)
- 1 egg (or egg substitute)
- 1 teaspoon vanilla extract
- Cooking spray or a small amount of olive oil for greasing the baking dish

Instructions:

1. Preheat your oven to 350°F (175°C) and grease an 8x8-inch baking dish with cooking spray or a small amount of olive oil.

2. In a mixing bowl, combine the rolled oats, chopped almonds, dried

cranberries, mixed berries, and ground cinnamon. Mix well.

3. In a separate bowl, whisk together the low-potassium milk substitute, honey (or sugar substitute), egg (or egg substitute), and vanilla extract until well combined.

4. Pour the wet mixture over the dry oat mixture and stir to combine.

5. Transfer the oatmeal mixture into the greased baking dish, spreading it evenly.

6. Bake in the preheated oven for about 30-35 minutes or until the top is golden brown, and the oatmeal is set.

7. Remove the baked oatmeal from the oven and allow it to cool for a few minutes before serving.

8. Cut into squares and serve warm.

This Baked Oatmeal with Berries is a kidney-friendly breakfast option that's rich in fiber, vitamins, and minerals. It provides a satisfying and nutritious start to your day while adhering to dietary restrictions for kidney disease. Adjust ingredients and portion sizes based on your specific dietary needs and recommendations from your healthcare provider or dietitian.

Poached eggs with Greens and Avocado

Ingredients:

- 2 large eggs
- 2 cups fresh spinach or kale (chopped, low in potassium)
- 1/2 ripe avocado, sliced
- 1 teaspoon olive oil
- Salt and pepper to taste
- 1 tablespoon lemon juice (optional)

Instructions:

1. Fill a saucepan with water, about 2-3 inches deep, and bring it to a gentle simmer over medium-low heat. Add a splash of white vinegar (about 1-2 tablespoons) to the water; this helps the egg whites coagulate more easily during poaching.

2. While the water is heating, heat the olive oil in a separate pan over medium heat. Add the chopped spinach or kale and sauté for 2-3 minutes until wilted. Season with a pinch of salt and pepper. If desired, add a squeeze of lemon juice for extra flavor.

3. Carefully crack each egg into a small bowl or ramekin, taking care not to break the yolks.

4. Create a gentle whirlpool in the simmering water by stirring it with a spoon. Carefully slide one egg into the center of the whirlpool, allowing the swirling water to envelop the egg white. This helps the egg white to set around the yolk.

5. Poach the egg for about 3-4 minutes for a runny yolk or longer for a firmer yolk. Use a slotted spoon to gently lift the poached egg from the water, allowing any excess water to drain. Repeat the poaching process with the second egg.

6. Place the sautéed greens on a serving plate. Top with sliced avocado.

7. Carefully place the poached eggs on top of the greens and avocado.

8. Season with a pinch of salt and pepper to taste.

9. Garnish with an additional squeeze of lemon juice, if desired.

10. Serve immediately, and enjoy your kidney-friendly Poached Eggs with Greens and Avocado!

This breakfast recipe is kidney-friendly, nutritious, and packed with protein, healthy fats, and leafy greens. Adjust ingredients and portion sizes based on your specific dietary restrictions and recommendations from your healthcare provider or dietitians.

Egg and Cheese Breakfast Burrito:

Ingredients:

For the Burrito:
- 2 large eggs
- 2 egg whites
- 1/4 cup low-phosphorus cheese (such as mozzarella or Swiss), grated
- 1/4 cup chopped bell peppers (choose low-potassium colors like green or yellow)
- 1/4 cup chopped spinach (or other low-potassium greens)
- 1/4 cup diced tomatoes (if your dietary restrictions allow)
- Salt and pepper to taste
- 1 whole-grain or low-sodium tortilla (check labels for kidney-friendliness)
- Cooking spray or a small amount of olive oil for the pan

For Garnish (optional):
- Salsa (choose a low-sodium variety if available)

- Fresh cilantro
- Avocado slices (in moderation, as avocado is higher in potassium)

Instructions:

1. In a bowl, whisk together the eggs and egg whites until well beaten. Season with a pinch of salt and pepper.

2. Heat a non-stick skillet over medium heat and lightly grease it with cooking spray or a small amount of olive oil.

3. Add the chopped bell peppers and spinach to the skillet and sauté for 2-3 minutes until they begin to soften.

4. Pour the beaten eggs over the sautéed vegetables and allow them to cook without stirring until the edges set.

5. Sprinkle the grated cheese evenly over the eggs.

6. Carefully fold one half of the egg mixture over the cheese side to form a half-moon shape.

7. Continue cooking for another 1-2 minutes until the cheese melts and the egg mixture is cooked through.

8. Warm the tortilla in the microwave for a few seconds or in a dry skillet for a minute to make it pliable.

9. Place the cooked egg and cheese mixture in the center of the tortilla.

10. Add diced tomatoes (if allowed) and any optional garnishes, such as salsa, fresh cilantro, or avocado slices.

11. Fold the sides of the tortilla over the filling, then roll it up from the bottom to create your breakfast burrito.

12. Serve your kidney-friendly Egg and Cheese Breakfast Burrito warm and enjoy!

This breakfast burrito is kidney-friendly, packed with protein, and customizable with your favorite low-potassium vegetables and garnishes.

Baked Apple with oats and walnut

Ingredients:

- 2 apples (choose low-potassium varieties if available)
- 1/4 cup rolled oats (choose low-sodium oats if available)
- 2 tablespoons chopped walnuts (unsalted)
- 1 tablespoon honey or a sugar substitute (if needed)
- 1/2 teaspoon ground cinnamon
- 1/2 teaspoon vanilla extract
- Cooking spray or a small amount of olive oil for greasing the baking dish

Instructions:

1. Preheat your oven to 375°F (190°C).

2. Wash and core the apples, leaving the bottoms intact. This creates a well in each apple to hold the filling.

3. In a bowl, combine the rolled oats, chopped walnuts, honey (or sugar substitute), ground cinnamon, and vanilla extract. Mix well.

4. Carefully stuff each apple with the oat and walnut mixture, pressing it gently into the well.

5. Place the stuffed apples in a baking dish lightly greased with cooking spray or a small amount of olive oil.

6. If desired, you can sprinkle a little extra cinnamon on top of the stuffed apples for added flavor.

7. Cover the baking dish with aluminum foil and bake in the preheated oven for approximately 25-30 minutes or until the apples are tender.

8. Remove the foil and bake for an additional 5-10 minutes or until the tops of the apples are lightly golden.

9. Carefully remove the baked apples from the oven and let them cool for a few minutes.

10. Serve your kidney-friendly Baked Apple with Oats and Walnuts warm, and enjoy!

This dessert or snack offers the sweetness of baked apples combined with the heartiness of oats and the crunch of walnuts. It's a kidney-friendly treat that's both satisfying and nutritious.

Avocado toast

Ingredients:

- 1 slice of whole-grain or low-sodium bread (choose a kidney-friendly option)
- 1/2 ripe avocado, peeled and pitted
- 1/4 teaspoon lemon juice (optional, to prevent browning)
- Salt and pepper to taste
- Optional toppings: sliced tomatoes, low-phosphorus cheese, fresh herbs, or a poached egg (if allowed)

Instructions:

1. Toast the slice of whole-grain or low-sodium bread until it's crispy and golden brown.

2. While the bread is toasting, mash the ripe avocado in a bowl with a fork until it reaches your desired level of smoothness.

3. If you'd like to prevent the avocado from browning, you can add a splash of lemon juice and mix it in.

4. Once the toast is ready, spread the mashed avocado evenly over the toasted bread.

5. Season the avocado toast with a pinch of salt and pepper to taste.

6. If you prefer, you can add additional toppings like sliced tomatoes, low-phosphorus cheese, fresh herbs, or a poached egg (if allowed by your dietary restrictions).

7. Serve your kidney-friendly Avocado Toast immediately, and enjoy!

This simple yet tasty recipe provides healthy fats, fiber, and nutrients from the avocado and whole-grain bread.

Fruit and nut garnola

Ingredients:

- 2 cups rolled oats (choose low-sodium oats if available)
- 1/2 cup chopped nuts (e.g., almonds, walnuts) (unsalted)
- 1/2 cup dried fruit (e.g., raisins, cranberries, apricots) (choose low-potassium options)
- 2 tablespoons honey or a sugar substitute (if needed)
- 2 tablespoons vegetable oil (or a kidney-friendly oil)
- 1/2 teaspoon vanilla extract
- 1/2 teaspoon ground cinnamon (optional)
- Pinch of salt (or a salt substitute)

Instructions:

1. Preheat your oven to 325°F (160°C) and line a baking sheet with parchment paper or a silicone baking mat.

2. In a large mixing bowl, combine the rolled oats, chopped nuts, and dried fruit. Mix well.

3. In a separate microwave-safe bowl or small saucepan, heat the honey (or sugar substitute), vegetable oil, vanilla extract, ground cinnamon (if using), and a pinch of salt. Heat until the mixture becomes smooth and well combined. This should take about 30 seconds in the microwave or a couple of minutes on the stovetop over low heat.

4. Pour the liquid mixture over the dry oat mixture in the large mixing bowl. Stir well to coat all the dry ingredients evenly with the liquid.

5. Spread the granola mixture evenly onto the prepared baking sheet.

6. Bake in the preheated oven for about 20-25 minutes, stirring every 10 minutes to ensure even browning. Keep a close eye on it to prevent over-baking.

7. Once the granola is golden brown and crisp, remove it from the oven and let it cool completely on the baking sheet.

8. Once cooled, break the granola into clusters and store it in an airtight container.

9. Serve your kidney-friendly Fruit and Nut Granola with low-potassium milk or yogurt, or enjoy it as a snack on its own.

This homemade granola allows you to control the ingredients to make it kidney-friendly while still enjoying the delicious combination of fruits and nuts.

Greek yoghourt parfait

Ingredients:

- 1 cup plain Greek yogurt (low in potassium)
- 1/2 cup fresh berries (e.g., strawberries, blueberries, raspberries)
- 1/4 cup chopped nuts (e.g., almonds, walnuts) (unsalted)
- 1-2 tablespoons honey or a sugar substitute (if needed)
- 1/4 teaspoon vanilla extract
- A sprinkle of ground cinnamon (optional)

Instructions:

1. In a small bowl, mix the Greek yogurt, vanilla extract, and honey (or sugar substitute) until well combined. Adjust the sweetness to your taste.

2. Start assembling the parfait by spooning a layer of the sweetened Greek yogurt into a serving glass or bowl.

3. Add a layer of fresh berries on top of the yogurt.

4. Sprinkle a portion of chopped nuts over the berries.

5. Repeat the layering process by adding more yogurt, berries, and nuts until you've filled your serving glass or bowl. The number of layers depends on your preference and portion size.

6. Optionally, sprinkle a little ground cinnamon on the top for added flavor.

7. Serve your kidney-friendly Greek Yogurt Parfait immediately and enjoy!

This parfait is not only kidney-friendly but also a nutritious and satisfying breakfast or snack option. It provides a good balance of protein, healthy fats, and fiber. Adjust the ingredients and portion sizes based on your specific dietary restrictions and recommendations from your healthcare provider or dietitian.

Sweet potato hush

Ingredients:

For the Hush Puppies:
- 1 cup mashed sweet potatoes (cooked and peeled)
- 1/2 cup cornmeal
- 1/4 cup all-purpose flour
- 1/4 cup finely chopped onion
- 1/4 cup finely chopped green bell pepper
- 1/4 cup finely chopped celery
- 1 egg
- 1/4 teaspoon baking soda
- 1/4 teaspoon salt (or a salt substitute)

- Cooking oil for frying (choose a kidney-friendly oil like canola or olive oil)

Instructions:

1. In a mixing bowl, combine the mashed sweet potatoes, cornmeal, all-purpose flour, chopped onion, chopped green bell pepper, and chopped celery. Mix well.

2. In a separate bowl, beat the egg and add it to the sweet potato mixture. Mix until everything is thoroughly combined.

3. Add the baking soda and salt (or salt substitute) to the mixture and stir until evenly distributed.

4. Heat about 1 inch of cooking oil in a deep skillet or frying pan over medium-high heat until it reaches 350°F (175°C).

5. Using a spoon or your hands, form small portions of the sweet potato mixture into balls or small patties.

6. Carefully place the sweet potato balls or patties into the hot oil and fry until they are golden brown, turning them occasionally to ensure even cooking. This should take about 3-4 minutes per side.

7. Once they are cooked and have a crispy exterior, use a slotted spoon to remove the hush puppies from the hot oil and place them on a plate lined with paper towels to drain any excess oil.

8. Serve your kidney-friendly sweet potato hush puppies warm as a delightful side dish or snack.

These sweet potato hush puppies are a flavorful and kidney-friendly twist on a classic Southern treat. Enjoy them as part of your balanced diet, adjusting ingredients and portion sizes based on your specific dietary restrictions and recommendations from your healthcare provider or dietitian.

Scrambled Egg Whites with Herbs

Ingredients:

- 4 egg whites
- 1-2 teaspoons chopped fresh herbs (e.g., parsley, chives, basil)
- Salt and pepper to taste
- Cooking spray or a small amount of olive oil (for greasing the pan)
- Optional: a splash of low-potassium milk substitute (such as almond or rice milk)

Instructions:

1. In a mixing bowl, whisk the egg whites until they become frothy. If desired, you can add a splash of low-potassium milk substitute to the egg whites for added creaminess.

2. Heat a non-stick skillet over medium heat and lightly grease it with cooking spray or a small amount of olive oil.

3. Pour the whisked egg whites into the heated skillet.

4. Allow the egg whites to cook undisturbed for a minute or so until they start to set around the edges.

5. Gently stir the egg whites with a spatula, pushing them from the edges towards the center of the skillet. Continue to cook, stirring occasionally, until the egg whites are mostly cooked but still slightly runny.

6. Just before they are fully cooked, sprinkle the chopped fresh herbs, salt, and pepper over the egg whites.

7. Continue to cook and stir for another minute or until the egg whites are fully cooked and fluffy.

8. Remove the scrambled egg whites with herbs from the skillet immediately to prevent overcooking.

9. Serve hot, garnished with extra fresh herbs if desired.

These scrambled egg whites with herbs are a light and nutritious breakfast or snack option.

They are low in potassium and high in protein, making them suitable for a kidney-friendly diet.

Chapter 5

Lunch

Lunch is a crucial meal that can be adapted to suit your dietary needs, including kidney-friendly options.

Kidney-Friendly Chicken Salad:

Ingredients:

- 4 oz grilled chicken breast (skinless and boneless), diced
- 1 cup mixed greens (e.g., lettuce, spinach)
- 1/4 cup cucumber, sliced
- 1/4 cup cherry tomatoes, halved
- 1/4 cup red bell pepper, chopped
- 1/4 cup red onion, finely sliced
- 2 tablespoons low-phosphorus salad dressing (choose a kidney-friendly option)
- 1 tablespoon chopped fresh herbs (e.g., parsley, basil)
- Salt and pepper to taste

Instructions:

1. Start by grilling or baking the chicken breast until fully cooked. Dice the chicken into bite-sized pieces.

2. In a large bowl, combine the mixed greens, cucumber slices, halved cherry tomatoes, chopped red bell pepper, and finely sliced red onion.

3. Add the diced chicken to the salad mixture.

4. Drizzle the low-phosphorus salad dressing over the salad ingredients and toss gently to coat. Adjust the amount of dressing to your taste and dietary restrictions.

5. Sprinkle chopped fresh herbs over the top for added flavor and freshness.

6. Season with salt and pepper to taste.

7. Serve your kidney-friendly Chicken Salad for a satisfying and nutritious lunch.

This salad provides a balance of protein, vegetables, and fresh flavors while adhering to kidney-friendly dietary recommendations.

Quinoa and Vegetable Stir-Fry:

Ingredients:

- 1/2 cup cooked quinoa (follow package instructions)
- 1 cup mixed stir-fry vegetables (e.g., bell peppers, broccoli, snap peas)
- 4 oz firm tofu or skinless, boneless chicken breast, diced
- 1-2 tablespoons low-sodium stir-fry sauce (choose a kidney-friendly option)
- 1 teaspoon sesame oil (optional)
- 1 tablespoon chopped green onions (for garnish)
- Cooking spray or a small amount of olive oil for stir-frying

Instructions:

1. Cook quinoa according to the package instructions and set aside.

2. Heat a skillet or wok over medium-high heat and lightly grease it with cooking spray or a small amount of olive oil.

3. Add diced tofu or chicken to the hot skillet and stir-fry until cooked through.

4. Remove the cooked protein from the skillet and set it aside.

5. In the same skillet, add the mixed stir-fry vegetables and stir-fry for 3-5 minutes until they become tender-crisp.

6. Return the cooked protein to the skillet with the vegetables.

7. Add cooked quinoa, low-sodium stir-fry sauce, and sesame oil (if using) to the skillet. Stir-fry for an additional 2-3 minutes to heat everything through and combine flavors.

8. Garnish with chopped green onions.

9. Serve your kidney-friendly Quinoa and Vegetable Stir-Fry for a wholesome and protein-rich lunch.

Turkey and Avocado Wrap:

Ingredients:

- 2-3 slices of low-sodium deli turkey breast
- 1 small whole-grain or low-sodium tortilla
- 1/4 avocado, sliced (in moderation, as avocado is higher in potassium)
- 1/4 cup mixed greens (e.g., lettuce, spinach)
- 1 tablespoon low-phosphorus or kidney-friendly mayo (if desired)
- 1/2 teaspoon Dijon mustard (optional)
- Salt and pepper to taste

Instructions:
1. Lay the whole-grain or low-sodium tortilla flat on a clean surface.

2. Spread low-phosphorus or kidney-friendly mayo (if using) and Dijon mustard (if desired) evenly over the tortilla.

3. Arrange the slices of low-sodium deli turkey breast on top of the tortilla.

4. Place sliced avocado and mixed greens on top of the turkey slices.

5. Season with a pinch of salt and pepper to taste.

6. Carefully roll up the tortilla, tucking in the sides to create a wrap.

7. Slice the wrap in half diagonally for easier handling.

8. Serve your kidney-friendly Turkey and Avocado Wrap for a satisfying and portable lunch option.

Lentil and Vegetable Soup:

Ingredients:

- 1 cup cooked lentils (low in phosphorus)
- 1 cup mixed vegetables (e.g., carrots, celery, green beans)
- 1/4 cup diced onions
- 1 clove garlic, minced
- 4 cups low-sodium vegetable broth
- 1/2 teaspoon dried thyme
- Salt and pepper to taste

- Chopped fresh parsley for garnish (optional)

Instructions:

1. In a soup pot, sauté the diced onions and minced garlic until they become fragrant.

2. Add the mixed vegetables and cook for a few minutes.

3. Pour in the low-sodium vegetable broth and bring the mixture to a boil.

4. Reduce the heat, add cooked lentils, dried thyme, salt, and pepper.

5. Simmer the soup for about 15-20 minutes until the vegetables are tender.

6. Serve your kidney-friendly Lentil and Vegetable Soup hot, garnished with chopped fresh parsley if desired.

Tuna Salad Lettuce Wraps:

Ingredients:

- 1 can of low-sodium tuna in water, drained
- 1-2 tablespoons low-phosphorus or kidney-friendly mayo (if desired)
- 1 teaspoon Dijon mustard (optional)
- 1/4 cup diced celery
- 1/4 cup diced red bell pepper
- 1-2 large lettuce leaves (e.g., iceberg or Romaine)
- Sliced cucumbers (for garnish)
- Salt and pepper to taste

Instructions:

1. In a bowl, combine the drained tuna, low-phosphorus mayo (if using), Dijon mustard (if desired), diced celery, and diced red bell pepper. Mix well.

2. Season the tuna salad with a pinch of salt and pepper to taste.

3. Place a large lettuce leaf flat on a clean surface.

4. Spoon the tuna salad mixture onto the lettuce leaf.

5. Roll the lettuce leaf around the tuna salad to create a wrap.

6. Serve your kidney-friendly Tuna Salad Lettuce Wraps with sliced cucumbers on the side.

Quinoa Salad with Chickpeas and Veggies:

Ingredients:

- 1 cup cooked quinoa (low in phosphorus)
- 1 cup canned chickpeas (drained and rinsed)
- 1/2 cup diced cucumber
- 1/2 cup cherry tomatoes, halved
- 1/4 cup diced red onion
- 1/4 cup chopped fresh parsley
- 2 tablespoons lemon juice
- 1 tablespoon olive oil (or a kidney-friendly oil)

- Salt and pepper to taste

Instructions:
1. In a large bowl, combine the cooked quinoa, canned chickpeas, diced cucumber, cherry tomatoes, diced red onion, and chopped fresh parsley.

2. In a separate small bowl, whisk together lemon juice and olive oil.

3. Drizzle the lemon juice and olive oil dressing over the quinoa salad mixture.

4. Season with salt and pepper to taste and toss everything together.

5. Serve your kidney-friendly Quinoa Salad with Chickpeas and Veggies cold as a refreshing and nutritious lunch option.

Veggie and Hummus Wrap:

Ingredients:

- 1 small whole-grain or low-sodium tortilla
- 1/4 cup hummus (choose a kidney-friendly option)
- 1/4 cup sliced cucumbers
- 1/4 cup shredded carrots
- 1/4 cup baby spinach leaves
- Salt and pepper to taste

Instructions:

1. Lay the whole-grain or low-sodium tortilla flat on a clean surface.

2. Spread a layer of hummus evenly over the tortilla.

3. Arrange sliced cucumbers, shredded carrots, and baby spinach leaves on top of the hummus.

4. Season with a pinch of salt and pepper to taste.

5. Carefully roll up the tortilla, tucking in the sides to create a wrap.

6. Slice the wrap in half diagonally for easier handling.

7. Serve your kidney-friendly Veggie and Hummus Wrap for a satisfying and portable lunch option.

Baked Salmon with Quinoa and Steamed Asparagus:

Ingredients:

- 4 oz salmon fillet
- 1/2 cup cooked quinoa (low in phosphorus)
- Steamed asparagus spears
- Lemon wedges for garnish
- Olive oil, salt, and pepper for seasoning

Instructions:
1. Preheat your oven to 375°F (190°C).

2. Season the salmon fillet with a drizzle of olive oil, salt, and pepper.

3. Place the salmon on a baking sheet and bake for about 15-20 minutes or until it flakes easily with a fork.

4. While the salmon is baking, steam the asparagus spears until tender.

5. Serve the baked salmon over a bed of cooked quinoa, with steamed asparagus on the side.

6. Garnish with lemon wedges for added flavor.

Black Bean and Vegetable Stir-Fry:

Ingredients:

- 1 cup cooked black beans (canned and rinsed or cooked from dry)
- 1 cup mixed stir-fry vegetables (e.g., bell peppers, broccoli, snap peas)
- 1/4 cup diced onions
- 1 clove garlic, minced
- 2 tablespoons low-sodium stir-fry sauce (choose a kidney-friendly option)
- 1 tablespoon vegetable oil (or a kidney-friendly oil)

- 1/2 teaspoon ground cumin (optional)
- Salt and pepper to taste

Instructions:
1. In a skillet or wok, heat the vegetable oil over medium-high heat.

2. Sauté the diced onions and minced garlic until they become fragrant.

3. Add the mixed stir-fry vegetables to the skillet and stir-fry for 3-5 minutes until they become tender-crisp.

4. Stir in the cooked black beans and ground cumin (if using).

5. Pour the low-sodium stir-fry sauce over the mixture and stir-fry for an additional 2-3 minutes to combine flavors.

6. Season with salt and pepper to taste.

7. Serve your kidney-friendly Black Bean and Vegetable Stir-Fry as a flavorful and protein-rich lunch.

Turkey and Veggie Kabobs:

Ingredients:

- 4 oz low-sodium turkey breast, cut into chunks
- Assorted low-potassium vegetables (e.g., zucchini, bell peppers, cherry tomatoes)
- Olive oil, lemon juice, and your choice of herbs/spices for marinade (choose kidney-friendly options)
- Wooden skewers, soaked in water

Instructions:
1. In a bowl, combine olive oil, lemon juice, and your choice of herbs or spices for a marinade. Mix well.

2. Thread the turkey chunks and assorted vegetables onto the soaked wooden skewers.

3. Brush the marinade over the kabobs.

4. Grill or broil the turkey and vegetable kabobs until the turkey is cooked through and the vegetables are tender.

5. Serve your kidney-friendly Turkey and Veggie Kabobs with a side salad or kidney-friendly dipping sauce if desired.

Eggplant and Tomato Stuffed Bell Peppers:

Ingredients:

- 2 bell peppers (choose low-potassium colors like green or yellow)
- 1 small eggplant, diced
- 1/2 cup diced tomatoes (if your dietary restrictions allow)
- 1/4 cup diced onions
- 1 clove garlic, minced
- 2 tablespoons kidney-friendly olive oil
- Salt, pepper, and your choice of herbs/spices for seasoning

Instructions:
1. Preheat your oven to 375°F (190°C).

2. Cut the tops off the bell peppers and remove the seeds and membranes.

3. In a skillet, heat the kidney-friendly olive oil over medium heat.

4. Sauté the diced eggplant, diced tomatoes (if allowed), diced onions, and minced garlic until the vegetables are tender.

5. Season the mixture with salt, pepper, and your choice of herbs or spices.

6. Stuff the bell peppers with the cooked eggplant and tomato mixture.

7. Place the stuffed bell peppers in a baking dish and cover with foil.

8. Bake in the preheated oven for about 30-35 minutes or until the bell peppers are tender.

9. Serve your kidney-friendly Eggplant and Tomato Stuffed Bell Peppers as a flavorful and satisfying lunch.

These lunch ideas offer additional variety and kidney-friendly options for your meal planning.

Chapter 6

Flavorful Dinner Recipes

Here are some flavorful kidney-friendly dinner recipes:

Lemon Herb Baked Chicken:

Ingredients:

- 4 boneless, skinless chicken breasts
- 2 tablespoons lemon juice
- 2 tablespoons olive oil (or a kidney-friendly oil)
- 2 cloves garlic, minced
- 1 teaspoon dried oregano
- 1 teaspoon dried thyme
- Salt and pepper to taste
- Lemon slices and fresh herbs for garnish (optional)

Instructions:
1. Preheat your oven to 375°F (190°C).

2. In a bowl, whisk together lemon juice, olive oil, minced garlic, dried oregano, dried thyme, salt, and pepper.

3. Place the chicken breasts in a baking dish and pour the lemon herb mixture over them.

4. Bake in the preheated oven for approximately 25-30 minutes or until the chicken is cooked through and no longer pink in the center.

5. Garnish with lemon slices and fresh herbs if desired.

Spaghetti with Tomato Basil Sauce:

Ingredients:

- 8 oz whole-grain or low-sodium spaghetti
- 2 cups low-sodium tomato sauce
- 1/4 cup fresh basil leaves, chopped
- 2 cloves garlic, minced
- 1 tablespoon kidney-friendly olive oil
- Salt and pepper to taste
- Grated Parmesan cheese (in moderation, if allowed)

Instructions:

1. Cook the spaghetti according to package instructions, then drain and set aside.

2. In a skillet, heat the kidney-friendly olive oil over medium heat.

3. Sauté the minced garlic until fragrant.

4. Add the low-sodium tomato sauce and chopped basil to the skillet, and simmer for a few minutes.

5. Season with salt and pepper to taste.

6. Toss the cooked spaghetti with the tomato basil sauce.

7. Serve your kidney-friendly Spaghetti with Tomato Basil Sauce, garnished with grated Parmesan cheese if allowed.

Grilled Lemon Herb Salmon:

Ingredients:

- 4 salmon fillets
- 2 tablespoons lemon juice
- 2 tablespoons olive oil (or a kidney-friendly oil)
- 1 teaspoon dried dill
- 1 teaspoon dried rosemary
- Salt and pepper to taste
- Lemon wedges for garnish (optional)

Instructions:
1. Preheat your grill to medium-high heat.

2. In a bowl, whisk together lemon juice, olive oil, dried dill, dried rosemary, salt, and pepper.

3. Brush the lemon herb mixture onto both sides of the salmon fillets.

4. Grill the salmon for about 3-4 minutes per side or until it flakes easily with a fork.

5. Garnish with lemon wedges if desired.

Mediterranean Chickpea Salad:

Ingredients:

- 1 can (15 oz) low-sodium chickpeas, drained and rinsed
- 1 cucumber, diced
- 1 cup cherry tomatoes, halved
- 1/4 cup red onion, finely chopped
- 1/4 cup fresh parsley, chopped
- 1/4 cup kidney-friendly olive oil
- 2 tablespoons lemon juice
- 1 clove garlic, minced
- Salt and pepper to taste
- Feta cheese (optional, in moderation, if allowed)

Instructions:
1. In a large bowl, combine chickpeas, diced cucumber, cherry tomatoes, chopped red onion, and fresh parsley.

2. In a separate small bowl, whisk together kidney-friendly olive oil, lemon juice, minced garlic, salt, and pepper.

3. Pour the dressing over the salad mixture and toss to combine.

4. If desired, top with crumbled feta cheese (in moderation).

5. Serve your kidney-friendly Mediterranean Chickpea Salad as a refreshing and satisfying dinner.

Baked Herb-Crusted Tilapia:

Ingredients:

- 4 tilapia fillets
- 2 tablespoons kidney-friendly olive oil
- 2 cloves garlic, minced
- 1/4 cup fresh breadcrumbs (from low-phosphorus bread)
- 2 tablespoons fresh parsley, chopped
- 1/2 teaspoon dried thyme
- 1/2 teaspoon dried oregano
- Salt and pepper to taste
- Lemon wedges for garnish (optional)

Instructions:

1. Preheat your oven to 400°F (200°C).

2. In a bowl, combine fresh breadcrumbs, chopped fresh parsley, dried thyme, dried oregano, salt, and pepper.

3. Brush the tilapia fillets with kidney-friendly olive oil and minced garlic.

4. Coat the tilapia fillets with the breadcrumb mixture, pressing it gently to adhere.

5. Place the coated tilapia fillets on a baking sheet.

6. Bake in the preheated oven for approximately 15-20 minutes or until the tilapia is cooked through and the crust is golden brown.

Garnish with lemon wedges if desired.

Stir-Fried Tofu with Vegetables:

Ingredients:

- 8 oz firm tofu, cubed
- 2 cups mixed stir-fry vegetables (e.g., broccoli, bell peppers, snow peas)
- 2 tablespoons low-sodium stir-fry sauce (choose a kidney-friendly option)
- 1 tablespoon kidney-friendly oil (e.g., canola or safflower oil)
- 1 clove garlic, minced
- 1/2 teaspoon grated ginger
- Salt and pepper to taste

Instructions:

1. In a wok or skillet, heat the kidney-friendly oil over medium-high heat.

2. Add the cubed tofu and stir-fry until it's lightly browned on all sides. Remove the tofu from the skillet and set it aside.

3. In the same skillet, add minced garlic and grated ginger. Sauté until fragrant.

4. Add the mixed stir-fry vegetables and stir-fry for 3-5 minutes or until they become tender-crisp.

5. Return the cooked tofu to the skillet.

6. Pour the low-sodium stir-fry sauce over the mixture and stir-fry for an additional 2-3 minutes to combine flavors.

7. Season with salt and pepper to taste.

8. Serve your kidney-friendly Stir-Fried Tofu with Vegetables as a protein-rich and flavorful dinner.

Roasted Vegetable and Quinoa Bowl:

Ingredients:

- 1 cup cooked quinoa (low in phosphorus)
- Assorted roasted vegetables (e.g., bell peppers, zucchini, carrots)
- 2 tablespoons kidney-friendly olive oil
- 1 teaspoon dried thyme
- Salt and pepper to taste

- Balsamic vinegar (optional, for drizzling)

Instructions:
1. Preheat your oven to 425°F (220°C).

2. Toss assorted vegetables with kidney-friendly olive oil, dried thyme, salt, and pepper.

3. Spread the seasoned vegetables in a single layer on a baking sheet.

4. Roast in the preheated oven for approximately 20-25 minutes or until the vegetables are tender and slightly caramelized.

5. Serve the roasted vegetables over cooked quinoa and drizzle with balsamic vinegar if desired.

These dinner recipes offer a variety of flavors and ingredients while adhering to kidney-friendly dietary guidelines.

Cilantro Lime Shrimp Tacos:

Ingredients:

- 8 oz shrimp, peeled and deveined
- 1 tablespoon kidney-friendly olive oil
- 1 clove garlic, minced
- Juice of 1 lime
- 2 tablespoons fresh cilantro, chopped
- Salt and pepper to taste
- 4 small whole-grain or low-sodium tortillas
- Sliced cabbage or lettuce, diced tomatoes, and low-phosphorus sour cream (optional, for toppings)

Instructions:
1. In a bowl, combine kidney-friendly olive oil, minced garlic, lime juice, chopped cilantro, salt, and pepper.

2. Toss the shrimp in this mixture and let it marinate for about 15 minutes.

3. Heat a skillet over medium-high heat and cook the shrimp for 2-3 minutes on each side or until they turn pink and opaque.

4. Warm the tortillas in a dry skillet for a minute to make them pliable.

5. Fill the tortillas with cooked shrimp and your choice of toppings, such as sliced cabbage or lettuce, diced tomatoes, and low-phosphorus sour cream if allowed.

6. Serve your kidney-friendly Cilantro Lime Shrimp Tacos for a zesty and satisfying dinner.

Mediterranean Quinoa Salad with Grilled Chicken:

Ingredients:

- 4 oz grilled chicken breast, diced
- 1 cup cooked quinoa (low in phosphorus)
- 1/2 cucumber, diced
- 1/2 cup cherry tomatoes, halved
- 1/4 cup red onion, finely chopped
- 1/4 cup crumbled feta cheese (optional, in moderation)
- 2 tablespoons kidney-friendly olive oil
- 2 tablespoons lemon juice
- 1 teaspoon dried oregano

- Salt and pepper to taste
- Kalamata olives (optional, in moderation)

Instructions:

1. In a bowl, combine diced grilled chicken, cooked quinoa, diced cucumber, halved cherry tomatoes, finely chopped red onion, and crumbled feta cheese (if using).

2. In a separate small bowl, whisk together kidney-friendly olive oil, lemon juice, dried oregano, salt, and pepper.

3. Pour the dressing over the salad mixture and toss to combine.

4. If desired, add Kalamata olives (in moderation) for extra Mediterranean flavor.

5. Serve your kidney-friendly Mediterranean Quinoa Salad with Grilled Chicken as a protein-rich and flavorful dinner.

Vegetarian Eggplant Parmesan:

Ingredients:

- 1 medium eggplant, sliced into rounds
- 1 cup low-sodium tomato sauce
- 1/4 cup shredded low-phosphorus mozzarella cheese
- 2 tablespoons grated Parmesan cheese (optional, in moderation)
- 1/2 teaspoon dried basil
- 1/2 teaspoon dried oregano
- Salt and pepper to taste
- Fresh basil leaves for garnish (optional)

Instructions:
1. Preheat your oven to 375°F (190°C).

2. Season eggplant slices with salt and pepper, then grill or bake them until tender (about 10-15 minutes).

3. In a baking dish, layer grilled eggplant slices with low-sodium tomato sauce, shredded mozzarella cheese, dried basil, dried oregano, and grated Parmesan cheese (if using).

4. Repeat the layers until all ingredients are used.

5. Bake in the preheated oven for approximately 20-25 minutes or until the cheese is bubbly and golden brown.

6. Garnish with fresh basil leaves if desired.

These dinner recipes offer a variety of flavors and options while following kidney-friendly dietary recommendations. Adjust ingredients and portion sizes based on your specific dietary needs and recommendations from your healthcare provider or dietitian. Enjoy your flavorful and kidney-friendly dinners!

Chapter 7

Snacks and Appetizers

Here are lots of kidney friendly snacks and appetizers

Cucumber and Greek Yoghourt Dip:

Ingredients:

- 1 cucumber, peeled and diced
- 1 cup low-fat Greek yogurt
- 1 clove garlic, minced (optional)
- 1 tablespoon fresh dill, chopped
- Salt and pepper to taste
- Baby carrots or celery sticks for dipping

Instructions:

1. In a bowl, combine diced cucumber, low-fat Greek yogurt, minced garlic (if using), chopped fresh dill, salt, and pepper.

2. Mix well and refrigerate for a couple of hours to let the flavors meld.

3. Serve the cucumber and Greek yogurt dip with baby carrots or celery sticks for a refreshing and kidney-friendly snack.

Baked Sweet Potato Fries:

Ingredients:

- 2 medium sweet potatoes
- 1-2 tablespoons kidney-friendly olive oil
- 1/2 teaspoon paprika
- 1/2 teaspoon garlic powder
- Salt and pepper to taste

Instructions:
1. Preheat your oven to 425°F (220°C).

2. Peel the sweet potatoes and cut them into thin fries or wedges.

3. Toss the sweet potato fries with kidney-friendly olive oil, paprika, garlic powder, salt, and pepper in a bowl.

4. Spread the seasoned sweet potato fries in a single layer on a baking sheet.

5. Bake in the preheated oven for approximately 25-30 minutes or until the fries are crispy and golden brown.

6. Serve your kidney-friendly Baked Sweet Potato Fries as a delicious and nutritious snack.

Hummus and Veggie Platter:

Ingredients:

- Low-phosphorus or homemade hummus
- Sliced cucumber
- Baby carrots
- Bell pepper strips (e.g., red, green, or yellow)
- Cherry tomatoes
- Low-sodium or homemade pita chips (optional)

Instructions:
1. Arrange a variety of sliced vegetables and cherry tomatoes on a platter.

2. Serve with low-phosphorus or homemade hummus for dipping.

3. If desired, add low-sodium or homemade pita chips to the platter.

4. Enjoy your kidney-friendly Hummus and Veggie Platter as a satisfying and nutritious snack or appetizer.

Sliced Apple with Almond Butter:

Ingredients:

- Sliced apple (choose low-potassium varieties if available)
- Almond butter (in moderation)

Instructions:

1. Slice an apple into wedges or rounds.

2. Serve with a small amount of almond butter for dipping.

3. This simple and kidney-friendly snack provides a balance of flavors and textures.

Cottage Cheese and Berries:

Ingredients:

- Low-fat cottage cheese
- Fresh berries (e.g., strawberries, blueberries, raspberries)

Instructions:

1. Scoop a portion of low-fat cottage cheese into a bowl.

2. Top with fresh berries for a creamy and fruity kidney-friendly snack.

These snack and appetizer ideas offer a variety of flavors and textures while adhering to kidney-friendly dietary guidelines. Adjust ingredients and portion sizes based on your specific dietary needs and recommendations from your healthcare provider or dietitian. Enjoy your kidney-friendly snacks and appetizers!

Fresh Fruit Popsicles

Fresh fruit popsicles are a delightful and kidney-friendly treat, especially during hot weather. Here's a simple recipe for making homemade fresh fruit popsicles:

Ingredients:

- 2 cups fresh kidney-friendly fruits (e.g., berries, kiwi, melon, peaches)
- 1-2 tablespoons honey (optional, for sweetness)
- 1/2 cup water

Instructions:

1. Wash, peel (if necessary), and chop the fresh fruits into small pieces.

2. Place the chopped fruits in a blender or food processor.

3. If you prefer sweeter popsicles, add 1-2 tablespoons of honey to the blender.

4. Add 1/2 cup of water to help blend the fruits into a smooth puree. You can adjust the amount of water to achieve your desired consistency.

5. Blend the fruits until you have a smooth and creamy puree.

6. Taste the puree and adjust the sweetness if needed by adding more honey.

7. Pour the fruit puree into popsicle molds, leaving a little space at the top for expansion when freezing.

8. Insert popsicle sticks into each mold.

9. Freeze the popsicles for at least 4-6 hours or until they are completely frozen.

10. To remove the popsicles from the molds, briefly run them under warm water to loosen the popsicles.

11. Serve your homemade fresh fruit popsicles for a cool and refreshing kidney-friendly dessert or snack.

Feel free to customize these popsicles with your favorite kidney-friendly fruits, and you can experiment with different fruit combinations. Enjoy the natural sweetness of the fruits in this healthy and delicious treat!

Caprese Skewers:

Ingredients:

- Cherry tomatoes
- Fresh mozzarella cheese balls (bocconcini)
- Fresh basil leaves
- Kidney-friendly balsamic glaze
- Wooden skewers

Instructions:
1. Thread cherry tomatoes, mozzarella cheese balls, and fresh basil leaves onto wooden skewers in alternating layers.

2. Drizzle with kidney-friendly balsamic glaze for added flavor.

3. Serve your Caprese Skewers as a simple and elegant kidney-friendly appetizer.

Rice Cakes with Tuna Salad:

Ingredients:

- Low-sodium rice cakes
- 1 can of low-sodium tuna in water, drained and flaked
- Low-phosphorus mayonnaise or Greek yogurt (as a binder)
- Diced celery
- Diced red onion
- Chopped fresh parsley
- Salt and pepper to taste

Instructions:
1. In a bowl, combine drained and flaked tuna with low-phosphorus mayonnaise or Greek yogurt to bind the mixture.

2. Add diced celery, diced red onion, and chopped fresh parsley to the tuna mixture.

3. Season with salt and pepper to taste and mix well.

4. Spread the tuna salad onto low-sodium rice cakes for a satisfying and crunchy kidney-friendly snack.

Guacamole with Sliced Bell Peppers:

Ingredients:

- 2 ripe avocados
- 1 small tomato, diced (if your dietary restrictions allow)
- 1/4 cup diced red onion
- 1 clove garlic, minced
- Juice of 1 lime
- Salt and pepper to taste
- Sliced bell peppers (e.g., red, green, or yellow) for dipping

Instructions:
1. Cut the avocados in half, remove the pits, and scoop out the flesh into a bowl.

2. Mash the avocados with a fork until you achieve your desired guacamole consistency.

3. Add diced tomato (if allowed), diced red onion, minced garlic, lime juice, salt, and pepper to the mashed avocados. Mix well.

4. Serve your kidney-friendly Guacamole with Sliced Bell Peppers as a nutritious and flavorful snack or appetizer.

These snack and appetizer ideas offer a variety of flavors and textures while following kidney-friendly dietary recommendations. Adjust ingredients and portion sizes based on your specific dietary needs and recommendations from your healthcare provider or dietitian. Enjoy your kidney-friendly snacks and appetizers!

Chapter 8
Smoothie

Of course! Smoothies are versatile and can be customized to your taste. Here's a basic smoothie recipe that you can adapt and modify as you like:

Basic Smoothie Recipe:

Ingredients:
- 1 cup of your choice of liquid (water, milk, almond milk, coconut water, etc.)
- 1/2 cup of frozen fruit (berries, banana, mango, etc.)
- 1/2 cup of fresh fruit (optional for extra freshness)
- 1/2 cup of Greek yogurt or a dairy-free alternative
- 1 tablespoon of honey or maple syrup for sweetness (optional)
- Ice cubes (optional, for a colder and thicker texture)

Instructions:
1. Add the liquid to your blender first.
2. Add the frozen fruit, fresh fruit, and yogurt.

3. If you want extra sweetness, add honey or maple syrup.

4. If you prefer a thicker texture or want to make it colder, add some ice cubes.

5. Blend everything until smooth and creamy.

6. Taste the smoothie and adjust sweetness or consistency if needed by adding more fruit, liquid, or sweetener.

7. Pour into a glass and enjoy your customized smoothie!

Feel free to experiment with different fruits, greens (like spinach or kale), protein powder, nut butter, or spices (like cinnamon) to create your perfect smoothie.

Certainly! Here are five more delicious smoothie ideas:

1. Tropical Delight Smoothie:
   - 1 cup coconut milk
   - 1/2 cup pineapple chunks (fresh or frozen)
   - 1/2 cup mango chunks (fresh or frozen)
   - 1 banana
   - 1/2 cup Greek yogurt (or coconut yogurt for a dairy-free option)

2. Green Energy Boost Smoothie:
   - 1 cup spinach leaves
   - 1/2 avocado
   - 1/2 cup green apple slices
   - 1/2 cup cucumber slices
   - 1 tablespoon honey (optional)

3. Chocolate Peanut Butter Protein Smoothie:
   - 1 cup almond milk
   - 2 tablespoons cocoa powder
   - 2 tablespoons peanut butter
   - 1 banana
   - 1 scoop of your favorite protein powder

4. Berry Blast Antioxidant Smoothie:
   - 1 cup mixed berries (strawberries, blueberries, raspberries)
   - 1/2 cup Greek yogurt
   - 1/2 cup orange juice
   - 1 tablespoon honey

5. Minty Watermelon Cooler:
   - 2 cups fresh watermelon chunks
   - 1/4 cup fresh mint leaves
   - 1/2 cup coconut water
   - 1 tablespoon lime juice
   - Ice cubes (optional)

6. Peachy Keen Smoothie:
   - 1 cup sliced peaches (fresh or frozen)
   - 1/2 cup plain Greek yogurt
   - 1/2 cup orange juice
   - 1/2 banana
   - A dash of cinnamon (optional)

7. Protein-Packed Almond Joy Smoothie:
   - 1 cup almond milk
   - 1/4 cup unsweetened shredded coconut
   - 1 tablespoon cocoa powder
   - 2 tablespoons almond butter
   - 1 scoop chocolate protein powder
   - 1/2 banana

These smoothies should provide a variety of flavors and options to enjoy. Customize them to your liking and dietary preferences!

Chapter 8

Desserts and Treats

Here are a few dessert and treat ideas:

1. Fruit Salad with Honey-Lime Drizzle:
   - Toss together a variety of fresh fruits like strawberries, kiwi, pineapple, and grapes.
   - Drizzle with a mixture of honey and freshly squeezed lime juice for a sweet and tangy treat.

2. Baked Apples with Cinnamon and Oats:
   - Core and slice apples, then toss with cinnamon and a sprinkle of oats.
   - Bake until tender for a warm and comforting dessert.

3. Chia Seed Pudding:
   - Mix chia seeds with your choice of milk (e.g., almond, coconut, or regular) and a sweetener like honey or maple syrup.
   - Refrigerate until it thickens, and top with fresh berries or nuts.

4. Frozen Banana Bites:

- Slice bananas into coins, dip them in yogurt or melted dark chocolate, and freeze for a cool treat.

5. Greek Yoghourt Parfait:

- Layer Greek yoghourt with granola and fresh berries for a satisfying and healthy dessert.

6. Oatmeal Raisin Cookies (with reduced sugar):

- Make classic oatmeal raisin cookies with less sugar for a guilt-free indulgence.

7. Avocado Chocolate Mousse:

- Blend ripe avocados with cocoa powder, honey, and a touch of vanilla extract for a creamy chocolate mousse.

8. Mixed Berry Sorbet:

- Puree mixed berries (e.g., strawberries, blueberries, and raspberries) with a bit of honey or agave syrup, then freeze for a refreshing sorbet.

9. Pumpkin Spice Energy Bites:

- Mix canned pumpkin, oats, almond butter, honey, and pumpkin spice, then roll into bite-sized balls for a fall-inspired treat.

10. **Yogurt-Dipped Strawberries:**
   - Dip fresh strawberries in Greek yogurt and freeze for a sweet and creamy snack.

Remember to adapt these recipes to your dietary needs and preferences, and enjoy these desserts and treats in moderation.

Satisfying Your Sweet Tooth

Low-Phosphorus Fruit Sorbet Recipe:

Ingredients:
- 2 cups of low-phosphorus fruits (such as apples, pears, or berries)
- 1/4 cup of water
- 2 tablespoons of lemon juice (freshly squeezed)
- 1/4 cup of granulated sugar (or a sugar substitute suitable for your dietary needs)

Instructions:

1. Wash, peel (if necessary), and chop the low-phosphorus fruits into small pieces.

2. In a saucepan, combine the chopped fruit, water, and sugar.

3. Heat the mixture over medium-low heat, stirring occasionally, until the fruit becomes tender and the sugar dissolves, forming a syrup-like consistency. This should take about 10-15 minutes.

4. Remove the mixture from heat and let it cool for a few minutes.

5. Transfer the fruit mixture to a blender or food processor
.

6. Add the freshly squeezed lemon juice
.

7. Blend until the mixture is smooth and well combined.

8. Taste the mixture and adjust the sweetness or tartness by adding more sugar or lemon juice if needed.

9. Pour the sorbet mixture into an ice cream maker and churn according to the manufacturer's instructions until it reaches a sorbet-like consistency.

10. If you don't have an ice cream maker, you can transfer the mixture to a shallow container, cover it, and place it in the freezer. Stir the mixture every 30 minutes until it firms up (about 2-3 hours)
.

11. Once the sorbet has reached the desired consistency, serve it in small bowls or glasses, garnished with fresh fruit or mint leaves if desired.

This low-phosphorus fruit sorbet is a refreshing and kidney-friendly dessert option for those with dietary restrictions related to phosphorus intake. Always consult with a healthcare professional or dietitian to ensure it's suitable for your specific dietary needs.

Kidney-Friendly Chocolate Mousse Recipe:

Ingredients:
- 1 package (12-14 ounces) of silken tofu (firm or extra firm)
- 1/3 cup unsweetened cocoa powder
- 1/4 cup honey or a sugar substitute suitable for your dietary needs
- 1 teaspoon vanilla extract
- A pinch of salt
- 1/4 cup almond milk or any low-phosphorus milk alternative
- Fresh berries or mint leaves for garnish (optional)

Instructions:
1. Drain and rinse the silken tofu to remove excess liquid.

2. Place the drained tofu, unsweetened cocoa powder, honey (or sugar substitute), vanilla extract, and a pinch of salt in a blender or food processor.

3. Blend until the mixture is smooth and well combined

4. While blending, gradually add the almond milk (or your preferred low-phosphorus milk alternative) to achieve your desired mousse consistency. You may need more or less milk, so add it slowly until you reach the desired texture.

5. Taste the mousse and adjust the sweetness to your preference by adding more honey or sugar substitute if needed.

6. Once the mousse is smooth and sweetened to your liking, transfer it to serving bowls or glasses.

7. Refrigerate the mousse for at least 1-2 hours to allow it to chill and firm up.

8. Before serving, you can garnish each serving with fresh berries or mint leaves if desired.

This kidney-friendly chocolate mousse is rich and satisfying while being mindful of phosphorus content. Always consult with a healthcare professional or dietitian to ensure it's suitable for your specific dietary needs.

Baking with Renal-Friendly Flours

Baking with renal-friendly flours can be a great option for individuals with kidney disease who need to watch their phosphorus and potassium intake. Here are some renal-friendly flours and tips for baking with them:

1. White Rice Flour: White rice flour is generally low in phosphorus and potassium. It can be used as a substitute for wheat flour in most recipes. Keep in mind that it tends to produce drier baked goods, so you may need to adjust liquid content.

2. Sorghum Flour: Sorghum flour is a good alternative to wheat flour. It's naturally gluten-free and has lower phosphorus and potassium levels. It works well in cookies, muffins, and pancakes.

3. Oat Flour (Low Phosphorus): Oat flour can be made by grinding low-phosphorus oats. It's a

nutritious option with lower phosphorus levels compared to wheat flour. Use it in baking recipes for a hearty texture.

4. Tapioca Flour: Tapioca flour is low in phosphorus and potassium and can be used to improve the texture of gluten-free baked goods. It's often used in combination with other flours.

5. Cornstarch: Cornstarch is another low-phosphorus and low-potassium option. It's commonly used as a thickener in recipes but can also be used in baking to add tenderness to gluten-free goods.

6. Coconut Flour (in moderation): Coconut flour is relatively low in phosphorus but contains moderate potassium. Use it in moderation and blend it with other flours in recipes. It can absorb a lot of liquid, so you may need to adjust the recipe accordingly.

When baking with these flours, keep these general tips in mind:

- Experiment with flour blends: Mixing different renal-friendly flours can often yield the best results in terms of texture and flavor.

- Adjust liquid: Some renal-friendly flours may require more or less liquid than traditional wheat flour. Be prepared to adjust the liquid content in your recipes to achieve the desired consistency.

- Add binding agents: Xanthan gum or guar gum can be added to gluten-free flour blends to improve texture and binding in recipes like bread and cakes.

- Monitor portion sizes: Even renal-friendly flours can contain some level of phosphorus and potassium, so be mindful of portion sizes to stay within your dietary restrictions.

Consult with a registered dietitian or healthcare professional for personalized guidance and recommendations on baking with renal-friendly flours based on your specific dietary needs.

Chapter 9

Staying Hydrated without Overloading on Fluids

- Herbal Tea Selection

Selecting the right herbal teas can be a soothing and enjoyable way to stay hydrated while managing your fluid intake and considering your dietary restrictions. Here are some renal-friendly herbal tea options to consider:

1. Chamomile Tea: Chamomile tea is caffeine-free and known for its calming properties. It's a gentle choice that is unlikely to cause any issues with kidney health.

2. Peppermint Tea: Peppermint tea is caffeine-free and can help with digestion. It's typically low in potassium and safe for most kidney patients.

3. Hibiscus Tea: Hibiscus tea is naturally tart and can be a flavorful choice. It's usually low in potassium and is known for its potential to help manage blood pressure.

4. Ginger Tea: Ginger tea can be soothing for the stomach and digestion. It's typically low in potassium and phosphorus.

5. Lemon Balm Tea: Lemon balm tea has a mild, lemony flavor and is caffeine-free. It's often well-tolerated and considered safe for kidney health.

6. Nettle Leaf Tea: Nettle leaf tea is caffeine-free and is sometimes recommended for its potential to support kidney function. However, it's essential to consult with a healthcare provider before adding it to your routine, as it can interact with certain medications.

7. Rooibos Tea: Rooibos tea is a caffeine-free, South African herbal tea that is generally safe for kidney patients. It has a mild, slightly sweet flavor.

8. Cinnamon Tea: Cinnamon tea can add warmth and flavor without significant potassium or phosphorus content. It's suitable for many renal diets.

When selecting herbal teas, it's essential to check the ingredient labels, especially if you're following a strict dietary restriction for potassium or phosphorus. Additionally, consult with your healthcare provider or a registered dietitian to ensure that the herbal teas you choose align with your specific dietary needs and any potential interactions with medications or health conditions.

Homemade Electrolyte Drinks

homemade electrolyte drink variations to keep you hydrated:

1. Coconut Water Electrolyte Drink:
   - 2 cups of coconut water (a natural source of electrolytes)
   - A pinch of sea salt (for sodium)
   - 2 tablespoons of honey or agave syrup (for sweetness and carbohydrates)
   - A squeeze of lime or lemon juice (optional, for flavor)

2. Watermelon Electrolyte Cooler:
   - 2 cups of fresh watermelon chunks
   - 1/2 cup of coconut water (for potassium and hydration)
   - A pinch of salt (for sodium)
   - 1 tablespoon of honey (for sweetness)

3. Cucumber Mint Electrolyte Refresher:
   - 2 cups of water
   - 1/2 cucumber, thinly sliced (for hydration)
   - A handful of fresh mint leaves (for flavor)
   - 1 tablespoon of honey (for sweetness)
   - A pinch of salt (for sodium)

4. Ginger and Honey Electrolyte Elixir:

- 2 cups of water
- 1-2 tablespoons of freshly grated ginger (for digestion and flavor)
- 2 tablespoons of honey (for sweetness and carbohydrates)
- A pinch of salt (for sodium)

5. Pineapple and Basil Electrolyte Fusion:

- 2 cups of water
- 1/2 cup of pineapple chunks (for flavor and hydration)
- A few fresh basil leaves (for a unique taste)
- 1 tablespoon of honey or agave syrup (for sweetness)

6. Berry Blast Electrolyte Refresher:

- 2 cups of water
- 1/2 cup of mixed berries (strawberries, blueberries, raspberries)
- 1 tablespoon of honey (for sweetness)
- A pinch of salt (for sodium)
- A squeeze of lemon or lime juice (optional, for flavor)

7. Pomegranate Electrolyte Elixir:

- 2 cups of water

- 1/2 cup of pomegranate juice (for flavor and antioxidants)

- 1-2 tablespoons of honey (for sweetness)

- A pinch of salt (for sodium)

8. Mango and Basil Electrolyte Infusion:

- 2 cups of water

- 1/2 cup of fresh mango chunks (for flavor and potassium)

- A few fresh basil leaves (for a unique taste)

- 1 tablespoon of honey (for sweetness)

- A pinch of salt (for sodium)

9. Peach and Lavender Electrolyte Cooler:

- 2 cups of water

- 1/2 cup of sliced peaches (for flavor and hydration)

- A pinch of dried lavender buds (for a subtle floral note)

- 1 tablespoon of honey (for sweetness)

- A pinch of salt (for sodium)

10. Carrot and Ginger Electrolyte Boost:

- 2 cups of water

- 1/2 cup of carrot juice (for flavor and nutrients)

- 1-2 tablespoons of honey (for sweetness)
- 1/2 teaspoon of freshly grated ginger (for flavor and digestion)
- A pinch of salt (for sodium)

These additional homemade electrolyte drinks offer a wide range of flavors and benefits. Adjust the ingredients to your liking and dietary preferences, and enjoy staying hydrated while replenishing essential electrolytes.

Limiting High-Potassium Drinks

Limiting high-potassium drinks is essential for individuals with kidney disease or those on a low-potassium diet. Here are five types of drinks to be cautious of due to their high potassium content:

1. Orange Juice: Orange juice is known for its high potassium content. A small serving can contribute a significant amount of potassium, so it's generally best to limit or avoid it if you have kidney disease.

2. Tomato Juice: Tomato juice is another beverage high in potassium. It's often used as a

base for various cocktails, but it's not suitable for individuals with potassium restrictions.

3. Sports and Energy Drinks: Many sports and energy drinks contain added potassium, which can be harmful for those with kidney issues. Always check the labels for potassium content and opt for alternatives when possible.

4. Coconut Water: While coconut water is often marketed as a natural electrolyte drink, it can be high in potassium. If you're on a low-potassium diet, it's advisable to consume it in moderation.

5. Vegetable Juices: Some vegetable juices, such as beet juice and carrot juice, can contain moderate to high levels of potassium. Be cautious when consuming these and consider diluting them with water to reduce potassium concentration.

When managing your potassium intake, it's crucial to consult with a healthcare provider or registered dietitian to determine your specific dietary restrictions and recommendations.

Chapter 10

Exercise and Kidney Disease

Exercise can have several positive effects on kidney health, but it's essential to approach it carefully, especially if you have kidney disease. Here's how exercise can impact kidney health and some tips for incorporating it into your routine:

Benefits of Exercise for Kidney Health:

1. Improved Cardiovascular Health: Regular exercise can help maintain healthy blood pressure and reduce the risk of heart disease, which is essential for individuals with kidney disease.

2. Weight Management: Exercise can aid in weight control, which is crucial for managing kidney disease, as excess body weight can strain the kidneys.

3. Increased Insulin Sensitivity: Exercise can improve insulin sensitivity, helping manage blood sugar levels. This is particularly important for those with diabetes, a common cause of kidney disease.

4. Enhanced Blood Flow: Physical activity promotes better blood flow, which can benefit kidney function by ensuring an adequate supply of oxygen and nutrients.

5. Stress Reduction: Exercise can help reduce stress levels, which can indirectly benefit kidney health by minimizing the impact of stress-related hormones on the kidneys.

Exercise Tips for Individuals with Kidney Disease:

1. Consult Your Healthcare Provider: Before starting or intensifying an exercise routine, consult your healthcare provider, especially if you have advanced kidney disease. They can provide personalized recommendations based on your specific condition and limitations.

2. Choose Appropriate Activities: Low-impact exercises like walking, swimming, cycling, and gentle stretching are often suitable for individuals with kidney disease. Avoid high-impact activities that can put excessive strain on the kidneys.

3. Stay Hydrated: Maintain proper hydration during exercise, but be mindful of your fluid intake if you have fluid restrictions due to kidney disease.

4. Monitor Blood Pressure: If you have hypertension, monitor your blood pressure regularly, and ensure it's well-controlled during exercise.

5. Start Slowly: If you're new to exercise or haven't been active for a while, start slowly and gradually increase the intensity and duration of your workouts. This approach minimizes the risk of injury.

6. Listen to Your Body: Pay attention to how your body responds to exercise. If you experience discomfort, pain, or excessive

fatigue, stop and consult your healthcare provider.

7. Medication Management: If you're taking medications, discuss with your healthcare provider how exercise might affect them, and ensure you're following the recommended medication schedule.

8. Maintain a Balanced Diet: Proper nutrition is essential for kidney health. Combine regular exercise with a balanced diet to support overall well-being.

Remember that the type and amount of exercise you can safely do may vary depending on the stage and severity of your kidney disease. Your healthcare provider can provide the most appropriate guidance for your individual situation.

MEAL PLANNING EXAMPLE

Simple Meal planning

Creating a meal plan for someone with kidney disease involves managing protein, sodium, potassium, and phosphorus intake.

Breakfast:
- Oatmeal made with water, topped with sliced strawberries and a sprinkle of chopped almonds (low in phosphorus and potassium)
- Whole grain toast with a small amount of margarine or butter
- A small serving of apple juice (check for low potassium options)

Snack:
- A small handful of grapes or a pear (low potassium fruits)
- A slice of low-sodium cheese or a hard-boiled egg (for protein)

Lunch:
- Grilled chicken breast salad with mixed greens, cucumbers, and cherry tomatoes (watch portions of protein)

- Balsamic vinaigrette dressing on the side (low sodium)
- A small serving of cooked carrots or green beans (low potassium vegetables)

Snack:
- Greek yogurt with a drizzle of honey (low phosphorus)
- A few whole grain crackers

Dinner:
- Baked salmon with lemon and herbs (rich in omega-3s and protein)
- Quinoa pilaf with sautéed spinach and mushrooms (low potassium)
- Steamed asparagus spears (low phosphorus)
- A small slice of whole grain bread

Snack/Dessert:
- A small serving of vanilla pudding made with low-fat milk (watch portion size)
- Sliced peaches or pineapple (in moderation)

Remember to consult with a dietitian or healthcare provider to tailor the meal plan to specific dietary needs and medical conditions. Additionally, proper hydration is crucial, so encourage drinking plenty of water throughout the day unless otherwise advised by a healthcare professional.

Conclusion

Maintaining a Renal-Friendly Lifestyle

In conclusion, maintaining a renal-friendly lifestyle is essential for individuals with kidney disease. By focusing on dietary management, proper hydration, medication adherence, regular check-ups, physical activity, stress management, smoking cessation, limited alcohol consumption, and quality sleep, you can take proactive steps to support your kidney health.

It's important to remember that each person's journey with kidney disease is unique, and individualized care and guidance from healthcare professionals, especially nephrologists and dietitians, are crucial. By working closely with your healthcare team and making informed choices, you can enhance your quality of life and effectively manage kidney disease. Prioritizing your well-being through a renal-friendly lifestyle is a significant step towards a healthier future.

More tips to help you maintain a renal-friendly lifestyle:

1. Dietary Awareness: Pay attention to food labels and ingredients to make informed choices. Be vigilant about hidden sources of potassium, phosphorus, and sodium in processed foods and restaurant meals.

2. Portion Control: Watch portion sizes to prevent excessive intake of nutrients that need to be limited. Use measuring cups or a food scale if necessary to ensure accurate portioning.

3. Regular Lab Monitoring: Follow your healthcare provider's recommendations for regular blood tests and urine tests. These tests help monitor your kidney function and detect any changes or complications early.

4. Support Network: Connect with support groups or organizations specializing in kidney health. Sharing experiences and information with others who have kidney disease can

provide valuable insights and emotional support.

5. Educate Yourself: Continuously educate yourself about kidney disease, its management, and treatment options. Knowledge empowers you to make informed decisions about your health.

6. Meal Planning and Preparation: Plan your meals in advance and prepare renal-friendly dishes at home whenever possible. Cooking at home allows you to have better control over ingredients and portion sizes.

7. Medication Record: Maintain a record of your medications, including dosages and schedules. This helps ensure you don't miss doses and can provide this information in case of emergencies.

8. Stay Informed: Stay updated on the latest research and advancements in kidney health. Knowledge is a valuable tool in managing your condition.

9. Regular Communication: Keep an open line of communication with your healthcare team. Inform them of any changes in your health or medications promptly.

Remember that living with kidney disease is a journey that requires ongoing attention and commitment. By incorporating these additional tips into your renal-friendly lifestyle, you can proactively manage your condition and improve your overall well-being.